AF667345

RECENT ADVANCES IN PHYLOGENETICS

Edited by **Zubaida Yousaf**

Recent Advances in Phylogenetics
http://dx.doi.org/10.5772/intechopen.73406
Edited by Zubaida Yousaf

Contributors

Ogueri Nwaiwu, Samina Sarwar, Qudsia Firdous, Abdul Nasir Khalid, Eliane Evanovich, Dowiya Benjamin Nzawele, Amon P. Maerere, Cornel L. Rweyemamu, Paul Kusolwa, Antoine Kanyenga Lubobo

© The Editor(s) and the Author(s) 2019
The rights of the editor(s) and the author(s) have been asserted in accordance with the Copyright, Designs and Patents Act 1988. All rights to the book as a whole are reserved by INTECHOPEN LIMITED. The book as a whole (compilation) cannot be reproduced, distributed or used for commercial or non-commercial purposes without INTECHOPEN LIMITED's written permission. Enquiries concerning the use of the book should be directed to INTECHOPEN LIMITED rights and permissions department (permissions@intechopen.com).
Violations are liable to prosecution under the governing Copyright Law.

(cc) BY

Individual chapters of this publication are distributed under the terms of the Creative Commons Attribution 3.0 Unported License which permits commercial use, distribution and reproduction of the individual chapters, provided the original author(s) and source publication are appropriately acknowledged. If so indicated, certain images may not be included under the Creative Commons license. In such cases users will need to obtain permission from the license holder to reproduce the material. More details and guidelines concerning content reuse and adaptation can be found at http://www.intechopen.com/copyright-policy.html.

Notice
Statements and opinions expressed in the chapters are these of the individual contributors and not necessarily those of the editors or publisher. No responsibility is accepted for the accuracy of information contained in the published chapters. The publisher assumes no responsibility for any damage or injury to persons or property arising out of the use of any materials, instructions, methods or ideas contained in the book.

First published in London, United Kingdom, 2019 by IntechOpen
IntechOpen is the global imprint of INTECHOPEN LIMITED, registered in England and Wales, registration number: 11086078, The Shard, 25th floor, 32 London Bridge Street
London, SE19SG – United Kingdom
Printed in Croatia

British Library Cataloguing-in-Publication Data
A catalogue record for this book is available from the British Library

Additional hard copies can be obtained from orders@intechopen.com

Recent Advances in Phylogenetics, Edited by Zubaida Yousaf
p. cm.
Print ISBN 978-1-78985-889-1
Online ISBN 978-1-78985-890-7

We are IntechOpen,
the world's leading publisher of
Open Access books

Built by scientists, for scientists

4,100+
Open access books available

116,000+
International authors and editors

120M+
Downloads

151
Countries delivered to

Our authors are among the
Top 1%
most cited scientists

12.2%
Contributors from top 500 universities

WEB OF SCIENCE™

Selection of our books indexed in the Book Citation Index
in Web of Science™ Core Collection (BKCI)

Interested in publishing with us?
Contact book.department@intechopen.com

Numbers displayed above are based on latest data collected.
For more information visit www.intechopen.com

For EU product safety concerns:
IN TECH d.o.o., Prolaz Marije Krucifikse Kozulić 3, 51000 Rijeka, Croatia,
info@intechopen.com or visit our website at intechopen.com.

Meet the editor

Dr. Zubaida Yousaf is working as an associate professor in the Department of Botany, Lahore College for Women University, Lahore. She joined this institute in 2009 as an assistant professor. She got her postdoc from South China Botanical Garden, Guangzhou, China, in 2011, funded by TWAS-CAS. She has authored 45 research articles and 4 books and contributed 6 chapters in international editors' books. She has overseen more than 40 MS theses and supervised 5 PhD students.

Contents

Chapter 1 **Phylogenetics 1**
Eliane Barbosa Evanovich dos Santos

Chapter 2 **Phylogeny of Three Palmwine Yeasts Genera 25**
Ogueri Nwaiwu

Chapter 3 **Importance of Molecular and Phylogenetic Analyses for Identification of Basidiomycetes 43**
Samina Sarwar, Qudsia Firdous and Abdul Nasir Khalid

Chapter 4 **Genetic Diversity in Banana and Plantains Cultivars from Eastern DRC and Tanzania Using SSR and Morphological Markers, Their Phylogenetic Classification and Principal Components Analyses 59**
Dowiya Benjamin Nzawele, Antoine Kanyenga Lubolo, Paul M. Kusolwa, Cornel L. Rweyemamu and Amon P. Maerere

Chapter 1

Phylogenetics

Eliane Barbosa Evanovich dos Santos

Additional information is available at the end of the chapter

http://dx.doi.org/10.5772/intechopen.79422

Abstract

Describing the diversity of living beings has always instigated man. The classification proposed by Aristotle today seems naïve and unnatural, but it lasted from ancient Greece until the publication of the Linnaeus *Systema Naturae* in 1758. Although quite accurate, the taxonomic classification proposed by naturalist Carl Linnaeus did not consider the evolutionary relationships between living beings. This view, although prior to Charles Darwin, only gained deserved prominence after *On the Origin of Species*. Only in the twentieth century, a new area founded by Hennig, phylogenetic systematics was implemented, and with this, a series of useful methods in the construction of phylogenetic trees arose, as maximum parsimony, neighbor joining, UPGMA, maximum likelihood, and Bayesian inference. With the advancement of information technology, phylogenetic analyses have become more sophisticated and faster. The algorithms used in the analysis programs have become more complex and realistic, favoring the addition of substitution models. The application of these data and the greater facility in generating nucleotide and amino acid sequences allowed the comparison previously unimaginable, for example, between bacteria and eukaryotes. In this way, the history of the advances of phylogenetic knowledge is confused with the greater knowledge about the origin of life.

Keywords: evolution, phylogenetic systematics, phylogenetic tree, taxonomy, phylogenetic methods

1. Introduction

Different criteria of biological classification were created throughout history. Some are arbitrary and do little to reflect the evolutionary relationship between species, for example, the Aristotelian system. But not always reflecting the relations of relatives was a concern. Even the iconic classification suggested by Linnaeus was not intended to reflect this relationship (although it is very consistent with current taxonomic classification). Only with Darwin and

IntechOpen

© 2018 The Author(s). Licensee IntechOpen. This chapter is distributed under the terms of the Creative Commons Attribution License (http://creativecommons.org/licenses/by/3.0), which permits unrestricted use, distribution, and reproduction in any medium, provided the original work is properly cited.

his successors did common ancestry gain prominence and was accepted as a fundamental tool in taxonomic analysis through Hennig. The systematic phylogenetic title of the book of the German entomologist opened the door to a new way of looking at taxonomy through kinship relations. The proposal of this new taxonomy would, therefore, be an unequivocal way of understanding the evolutionary history of the species. We now know the various phylogenetic artifacts that may mask or hinder a robust phylogenetic hypothesis. But, computational advancement and new phylogenetic approaches are emerging, reducing the effects of these artifacts. This chapter makes a narrative review of the history and current advances in phylogeny. The analysis was conducted using PubMed (https://www.ncbi.nlm.nih.gov/pubmed/), Scopus (https://www.scopus.com), and Google Scholar (https://scholar.google.com/). The first part of the review describes succinctly the work of Anaximander, Aristotle, Carl Linnaeus, Peter Simon Pallas, Charles Darwin, and Willi Hennig; the second aspect is showing the phylogenetic methods and phylogenetic analysis programs, and the third focus presents the difference between gene tree and species and shows the criteria used in building of tree of life.

2. Phylogeny

> *"...the whole system of organic bodies may be well represented by the likeness of a tree that immediately from the root divides both the simplest plants and animals, [but they remain] variously contiguous as they advance up the trunk, Animals and Vegetables; those leading, from Mollusca advancing to Pisces, with great lateral branches of Insects sent out among themselves, from here to Amphibia; and at the extreme top of the tree the Quadrupeds are supported, Aves truly thrust out as an equally great lateral branch below the Quadrupeds. At the same time this image shows the animals to be neither continuous nor neighboring, but standing like a lone tree"* [1].

Biodiversity has always instigated man to explain its origin, define it, and classify it. The precursory attempts were from the Greeks Anaximander of Miletus (610–545 BC) and Aristotle (384–322 BC). Anaximander defended the proposal that living beings originated from water and underwent transformations over time [1]. The sun would be a catalyst for these changes and would have allowed the maturation and exit of a fish-like being from the water, giving rise to more complex creatures such as man [2, 3]. Aristotle developed one of the first animal classification systems based on different pluralistic criteria, which could be based on behavior, the way of life, development, mobility, etc. [4, 5]. It was a non-hierarchical system and admitted that the same animal classified into over one group. Von Lieven and Humar [6] performed an analysis on the zoological classification performed by Aristotle. They used 157 features used by the Greek and found 58 monophyletic groups, 29 of which were consistent with the groupings created by Aristotle. Therefore, Aristotle's classification was inaccurate but not arbitrary.

The Aristotelian system was accepted for almost 2000 years ago and was definitively replaced after the publication of the 10th edition of the Linnaeus *Systema Naturae* in 1758 by the Swedish naturalist Carl Linnaeus (1707–1778). The classification presented by Linnaeus was a landmark of zoological and botanical nomenclature, standardizing the classification systems in binomial and hierarchical [7]. The taxonomy presented by him presented the taxonomic levels of kingdom (divided in Animalia, Plantae, and Protista), phyla, classes, orders, families, genera, and species. For example, one of the fish studied by Aristotle in History of Animals, the kobios (or giant goby), according to the classification of Linnaeus, came to be called *Gobius cobitis*. In the Latinized name, *Gobius* corresponds to the genus, and cobius means the specific epithet.

http://dx.doi.org/10.5772/intechopen.79422

Linnaeus was a fixer, but admitted in his classification the similarity between man and apes, and described hybridization in plants and animals, a fact which, according to him, was contrary to the stability of divine creatures [8]. Although ancestry is a classificatory criterion by other naturalists, such as Peter Simon Pallas (1741–1811) and Carl Edward von Eichwald (1795–1876) before Charles Darwin, it only gained prominence in 1859 with the publishing of the book *On the Origin of Species* [9]. But it only merged after the apogee of the synthetic theory of evolution, a scientific theory that united the knowledge of Gregor Mendel and Charles Darwin and the principles of population genetics. The synthetic theory had a long maturation that began early in the twentieth century and gained popular visibility with the release of the book *Evolution: The Modern Synthesis* in 1942 by Julian Huxley.

The advance of evolutionary ideas brought to light the proposals of today's renowned German entomologist Willi Hennig (1913–1976). He proposed in 1950 in the book *Phylogenetic Systematics* (translated from German into English in 1966) that biological classifications based on genealogical relationships between organisms are natural and unequivocal, so it is a biological reference system [10, 11]. The taxonomy created by Linnaeus today could be called phenetic taxonomy or numerical taxonomy, while the *Phylogenetic Systematics* could also be called cladistic taxonomy. The phenetic taxonomy is based on common observable features that do not necessarily reflect the phylogenetic relationship between groups. It gained many followers in the 1950s and 1960s, with the arrival of biostatistical methods and numerical computing, and had as main representatives Peter Sneath (1923–2011) and Robert R. Sokal (1926–2012) [12].

2.1. Phylogenetic tree

The phylogenetic tree or cladogram presents the following elements: node, branch, clade, root, branch lengths, and topology. Node is the branch point in the tree; the branch represents the descendant and ancestry; a clade is the groups that include the commune and descendant; the root is the common ancestor between the clades. Topology is the branching pattern of the tree, and branch length corresponds to changes in the branches. The elements of the tree are shown in **Figure 1**.

The characteristics used in the phylogenetic trees can be classified in two ways: those shared by ancestry, that is, the homologies, and others not evolutionarily related but with an analog

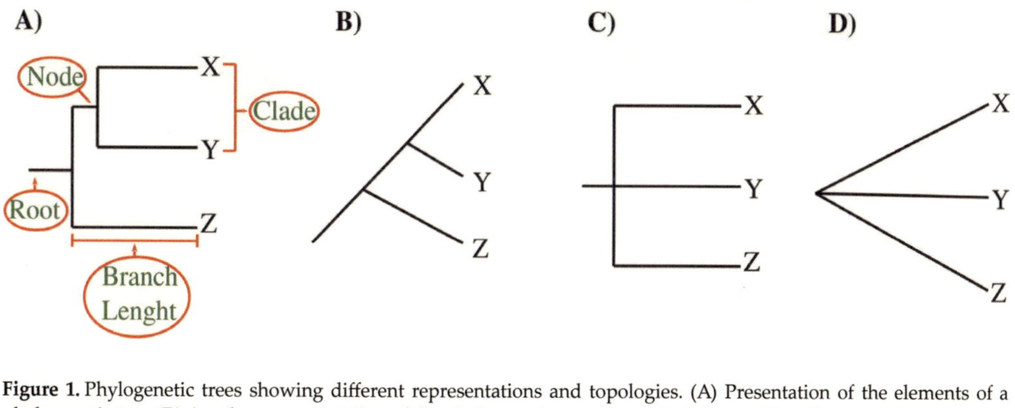

Figure 1. Phylogenetic trees showing different representations and topologies. (A) Presentation of the elements of a phylogenetic tree. (B) Another representation of the phylogenetic tree shown in A. Trees (C) and (D) are like each other and present topology that differs from trees A and B.

function called convergence or parallelism [13]. For example, homologies are present in species with recent common ancestors, as mammary glands and hairs present in mammals. The wings present in bats, birds, and insects are analogies. The comparison between analogy and homology is shown in **Figure 2**.

In a phylogenetic tree, the homologous characters are wanted. The convergences (also called homoplasy) may compromise the phylogenetic inference, although often present. After determining a homology, the next step to use it in a phylogeny is to determine its character state, to establish whether it derived from ancestral, that is, it is an apomorphy or plesiomorphy. One way to determine apomorphism and plesiomorphism is through character polarization by comparison with an external group. The out-group is a related taxon (i.e., a taxonomic unit) that one hopes to analyze [13]. For example, if the aim is to analyze the class Mammalia, it is interesting to have an out-group of another class of Amniota. If the target taxon is the primate, use as an out-group of another taxon from the superorder Euarchontoglires may be ideal. Once the out-group has defined, polarization can be made by comparing common traits to determine the apomorphies and plesiomorphies. The shared traits among the members of the target group are apomorphies, while those shared with the external group are plesiomorphies. A tree without an out-group is an unrooted tree, a tree in which the phylogenetic relationship between the branches is unclear (**Figure 3**). The tree of life, for example, is an unroot, since is not known the last universal common ancestor (LUCA).

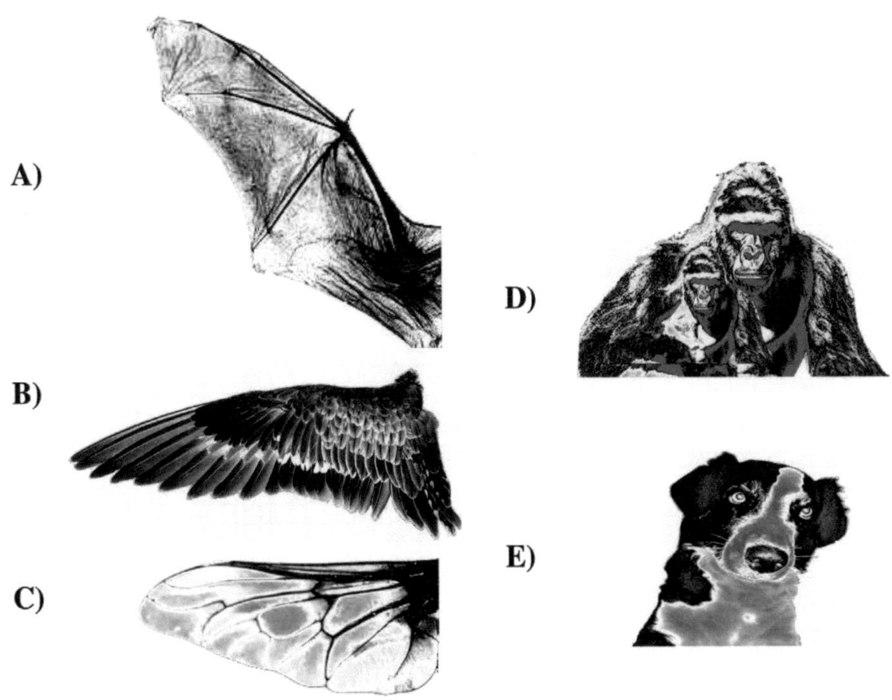

Figure 2. Difference between analogy and homology. In (A) is shown the wing of a bat, in (B) the wing of a bird, and (C) the wing of an insect. The three wings did not arise by common ancestry but by convergence or parallelism. The mammals (D) (gorilla) and (E) (dog) present homologies as mammary glands and hairs because they have a recent common ancestry.

http://dx.doi.org/10.5772/intechopen.79422

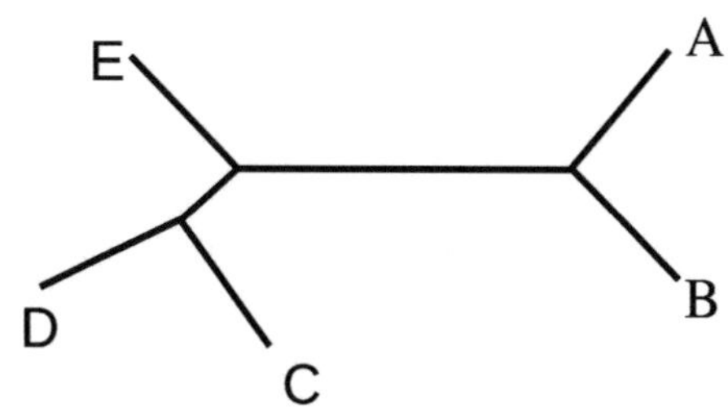

Figure 3. Representation of an unrooted tree. A, B, C, D, and E correspond to each of the taxa.

The apomorphies shared with the monophyletic group (a clade with all the ancestors and descendants) present a more recent common ancestor. Those apomorphies shared by two or more groups in a group are called synapomorphies [10, 13]. For example, having five digits is a synapomorphic trait of the modern tetrapods (the earliest tetrapods Acanthostega, Ichthyostega, and Tulerpeton presented more digits than the present species). Another type of apomorphism is the autapomorphies, specific characteristics of a group or taxon [13]. The plesiomorphy can be a symplesiomorphy that corresponds to when the ancestral characteristic is shared between certain clades [10, 13]. The different character states used in phylogeny are shown in **Figure 4**.

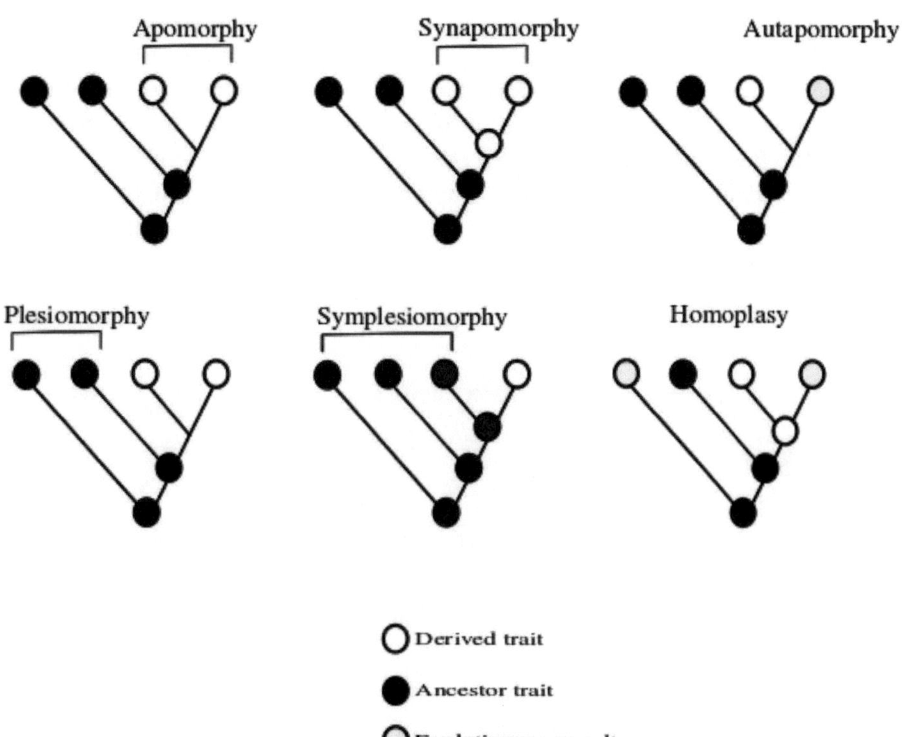

Figure 4. Types of characters used in phylogenetic trees. The different derived characters (apomorphy, synapomorphy, and autapomorphy) are shown in trees (A), (B), and (C). Meanwhile, the derived characters (plesiomorphy and symplesiomorphy) are shown in trees (D) and (E). Tree (F) presents the homoplasy, a convergence [13, 14].

2.2. Monophyletic, paraphyletic, and polyphyletic groups

Hennig assumed that phylogenetic relationships exist at different hierarchical levels, and the main role of phylogenetic systematics is to define the different degrees of kinship that can be in a phylogenetic tree [10]. One group that can be arranged in this tree is called a monophyletic group, which is defined by the author as "a group of species that contains all descendants of a single ancestral species" [10]. Within this context, species are reproductive communities isolated from others. The paraphyletic group exhibits some of its members in other groups, not monophyletic, as an example is Reptilia. It has Chondrichthyes (class formed by cartilaginous fishes) and Actinopterygii (superclass formed by ray-finned fishes). The second group presents a more recent common ancestry with Sarcopterygii (another superclass) but retained characteristics similar to those found in Chondrichthyes, such as gills. That is why Chondrichthyes and Actinopterygii often placed in the same group, but they are not. According to Hennig, the paraphyletic groups for being artificial should be abolished [10, 14]. The polyphyletic group also does not make up a natural group, and although they share common characteristics (by homoplasy), they do not have an immediate common ancestor. Both paraphyletic and polyphyletic groups produce uncertain phylogenies that are caused by a large number of homoplasies that can exceeds the amount of synapomorphies. Some fossil groups, due to the scarcity of data, may appear as paraphyletic or polyphyletic. Current groups, however, present a more robust classification because of the more sophisticated phylogenetic methods that use DNA or genome as the source of the data matrices. Hennig was right in wanting to abolish paraphyletic and polyphyletic groups, but it is not a trivial task. These groups are present even in more modern analyses based on data got by DNA sequencing. Some of these clusters result from a complex evolutionary history resulting from the exchange of genetic material between little related taxa. The horizontal transfer between bacteria can generate this evolutionary pattern of little clade containing possible polyphyletic and paraphyletic groups. But this matter will be treated more later. **Figure 5** shows the graphic representation of monophyletic, paraphyletic, and polyphyletic groups.

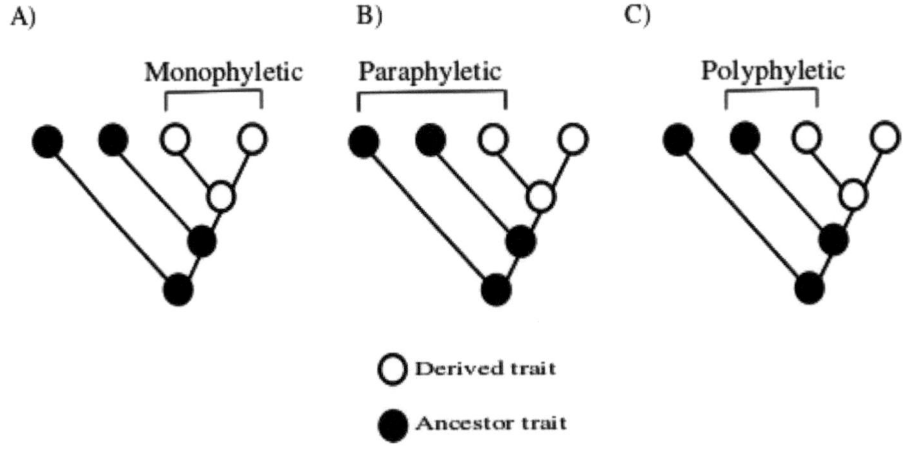

Figure 5. The phylogenetic tree shows the monophyletic, paraphyletic, and polyphyletic group. The monophyletic clade has only members with the same recent common ancestor (A), while the paraphyletic group has members in other groups (B) and the paraphyletic group (C).

http://dx.doi.org/10.5772/intechopen.79422

2.3. Phylogenetic inference methods

2.3.1. Parsimony methods

The maximum parsimony method was one of the first methods use for construction of phylogenetic trees. This method obeys Occam's razor—a principle created by William of Ockham (1285–1347). According to this idea, the simplest hypothesis would be the best since nature tends to the economy. To analyze the best phylogenetic hypothesis, it is necessary to assemble a data matrix based on derived ancestral characters got by the comparison between the taxa with the out-group. By convention, the ancestral state that is present in the out-group is represented by 0 (zero), and the derived state is by 1 (one). Besides this binary matrix, the algorithm also performs analyses with matrices based on alignments of DNA and amino acid sequences. In the matrix only, some characters parsed. **Figure 6** shows an array constructed from a short nucleotide sequence of four hypothetical taxa (X, Y, Z, and W). In it there are 10 characters, only those of sites 2, 5, and 6 are informative (at least 2 taxa have the same nucleotide), and site 10 appears homoplasic.

The inference by maximum parsimony is inconsistent when there is a high rate of mutation in certain branches. And also presents a great problem is to consider all the sites with an equal chance of change; however, this does not correspond to biological reality [15]. Nucleotides and amino acids present different chances of change, and this should be considered when assembling a phylogeny.

During DNA replication, the DNA polymerase enzyme can incorporate nucleotide mismatch. If this failure is not repaired, the nucleotide sequence will show mutations. Transitions are mutations of the purine for a purine (e.g., A → G or G → A) or a pyrimidine for a pyrimidine (e.g., C → T or T → C), while the transversion is the shift from purine for a pyrimidine or vice versa (e.g., A → C or T, G → C or T, C → A or G, T → A or G). The transversions require more complex change, so they are less common than the transitions. Under the position of the mutation in the codon (first or second, mainly), it may cause an amino acid change and may give in the protein structure.

Then, the maximum parsimony is unrealistic. For example, in **Figure 5A**, the sites 2 and 5 of the taxon Z have two transitions in 2C → T, 5 T → C base positions in relation to X and

A)

Taxa	DNA Sequence (Sites)									
	1	2	3	4	5	6	7	8	9	10
X	A	C	G	A	T	C	C	G	A	C
Y	A	C	G	G	T	C	C	G	A	T
Z	A	T	G	C	C	A	C	A	A	C
W	T	A	G	T	A	A	G	G	A	T

B)

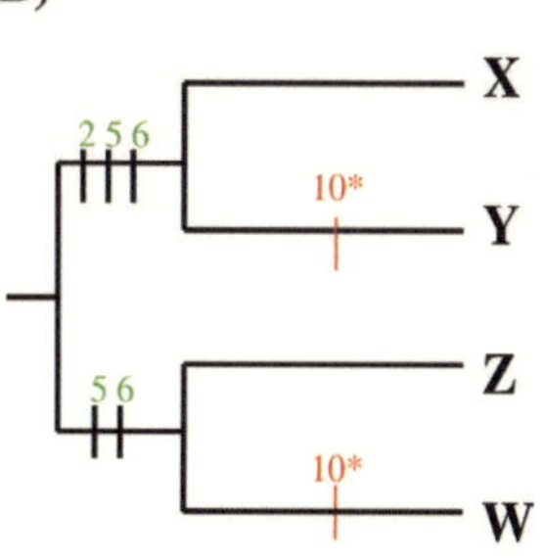

Figure 6. Simplified scheme of an array of nucleotide data characters (A) and phylogenetic tree assembled from data obtained from it (B). The sites highlighted in green in the matrix and tree correspond to the informational sites, and those in red is a supposed homoplasy site.

Y taxa. This may appear a clustering between the taxons X, Y, and Z. However, this clade is not formed due to the limitations of the method. The same problem can be observed in phylogenies built up from amino acid data. The amino acid exchanges with same physicochemical properties are not recognized by inference. Phylogenies based on maximum parsimony likewise present a major problem, the long-branch attraction (LBA), a phylogenetic artifact with high mutation rates forming erroneous groupings [16]. But, this does not mean that the maximum parsimony method will be abolished. It is even useful in analyses of conserved sequences, morphological and fossil data. In addition, the method has been optimized in different softwares [17–19].

2.3.2. *Distance methods*

The method infers the average number of changes per site between two rates. The total distance will be the division of the number of changes by the length of the sequence. In a sequence of 100 nucleotides, if the number of different bases between two sequences is 2, then the distance between them will be D = 0.02. The correction of this value is by the formula.

$$\textbf{Jukes - Cantor:dxy} = -(3/4)\ln(1\text{–}4/3D). \tag{1}$$

Dxy is the value of the correct distance between homologous sequences x and y, ln is the natural log (used to correct overlap of substitutions), and D is the observed distance between x and y. 3/4 and 4/3 reflect the nucleotides and have an equal chance of change. This formula is applied when the nucleotides have equal chances of change. Other more complex evolutionary models can also be assumed, such as the general time-reversible model (GTR), which assigns different probabilities for each type of change. Neighbor joining (NJ) method is the most used method, being fast. It uses the principle of parsimony or minimal evolution to find the best tree, based on the shortest length of the branches, with less evolutionary changes [20]. Although using the principle of parsimony, phylogenetic inference from NJ is more accurate, and together with unweighted pair group method with arithmetic mean (UPGMA), it is used in genomic analyses [21, 22].

2.3.3. *Maximum likelihood (ML)*

The maximum likelihood method was implemented by Anthony W. F. Edwards (1935-) and Luigi Luca Cavalli-Sforza (1922–2018) in the mid-1960s [23]. It is used to infer unknown parameters of a probability model in phylogeny analyses of different types of phylogenies and is able to estimate the length of the branches with a heuristic algorithm which is the phylogenetic tree that most likely to be generated from a given DNA sequence [24]. It can be defined by.

$$\mathbf{L = P(D \mid \theta).} \tag{2}$$

D corresponds to the probability of the dataset in a hypothesis θ. These hypotheses may be different parameters. The likelihood of each calculated nucleotide site and the total likelihood of the sequence are obtained from these data [24]. The probability of base substitution

http://dx.doi.org/10.5772/intechopen.79422

occurring at time t is simplified by Pij (t). i and j correspond to the states of the sites. The probability of i changing to state j at time t is represented by Pij (t). The states correspond to bases A, C, G, or T or S = {1, 2, 3, 4}. Mutations in the bases are called random variables in a stochastic process. PMF or probability mass function of a random variable X is given by the formula.

$$\mathbf{pX(x) = P(X = x).} \tag{3}$$

This formula is applied when mutations have equal possibilities of occurring in the DNA sequence. Then, 0.25 is the probability for each of the four nucleotides, and can be represented as: pX (1) = 0.25, pX (2) = 0.25, pX (3) = 0.25, and pX (4) = 0.25.

Because the current and future states are independent, it presents a process with Markov property, and if the variables pass from another state after a certain time t, then the substitution process can be considered continuous-time Markov process and may be represented by.

$$\mathbf{Pij = P(X(t+s) = j \mid X(s) = i).} \tag{4}$$

The rows representing i (current state) and j (future state) are shown in columns. Each Pij item of the matrix is the probability of the process Markov at a time t. The ergodic Markov process (aperiodic and positive recurrent) and time reversibility properties are also assumed during the likelihood analyses. It is, therefore, the final inference of the product of different events and parameters, which makes it exhaustive and demands a great computational time, but it creates a more realistic phylogenetic scenario, as it also allows to test the phylogenetic hypothesis within complex substitution models (e.g., Hasegawa, Kishino, and Yano (HKY), and general time-reversible (GTR), established as the specific program as ModelTest or jModelTest [25, 26]. These models allow us to evaluate how nucleotide sequences evolve and which model best describes them. The best evolutionary hypothesis is tested by likelihood ratio tests (LRTs). It is an important step of phylogenetic inference because although ML is less sensitive to LBA, it is not a free method of this artifact when the assumed evolutionary model is wrong [16, 27–30].

2.3.4. *Bayesian inference*

As the maximum likelihood, the Bayesian inference is also a probabilistic method. The method was developed by Thomas Bayes theorem (1701–1761) and consists of describing the probability of events based on a priori knowledge about the event. The theorem is described by the equation

$$\mathbf{P(A \mid B) = \frac{P(B \mid A)\, P(A)}{P(B)}.} \tag{5}$$

A and B are the events, and P (B) $\neq$ 0.

P (A) and P (B) are the a priori probabilities of events A and B;

P (A ∣ B) is the a posteriori probability of A conditioned to B;

and P (B ∣ A) is the a posteriori probability of B conditioned to A.

The method was applied to phylogeny only from 1990, but the initial idea was generated in 1967 by Cavalli-Sforza and Edwards who used it in the estimation of gene frequencies in human populations [31]. The improvement of the initial idea allowed its optimization and application to nucleotide sequences and also added other mathematical processes to phylogenetic parameters. Birth-death process is used as a model of speciation and extinction of a priori distributions of phylogeny and length of branches [32]. The model of nucleotide substitution is estimated by the continuous-time Markov process [32], while the substitution models and model parameter of the branches are inferred by maximum likelihood [33]. The distribution of a posteriori is obtained through the Bayes theorem and performed through some known data a priori (D) and unknown parameters θ, applied to the equation below [34]:

$$f(\theta \mid D) = \frac{1}{z} f(\theta) f(\theta \mid D). \tag{6}$$

f (θ | D) is called likelihood and z = ∫ f (θ)f (θ | D), normalizing constant.

The inference of the a posteriori distribution of phylogenies is performed with Markov chain Monte Carlo (MCMC) under the algorithm Metropolis-Hastings algorithm. The highest posterior probability is used to choose the best estimate [32, 33].

One of the problems of the method is to choose the optimal size to run the MCMC string to generate good later probabilities. If the value of the string is too low, the tendency is for the data to be large deviations and not realistic. In contrast, a long time can generate a very high computational time. One way to reverse this problem is to check the stationary phase (when the values a posteriori are stable) using different string sizes through programs such as R and Tracer; plotting the data will allow evaluating the consistency of the data [34]. In addition, some authors [35–37] point out that when a large database is analyzed by Bayesian inference the tree tends to present arbitrary polytomies (unresolved branches with more than two clades appearing at the same time) with auto values of posterior probability, but this problem is easily solved by modification in the Metropolis-Hastings algorithm so that a less-resolved topology is assumed [38]. With the use of the method, it is possible to analyze DNA data, amino acids, as well as morphological data [34].

2.4. Data resampling approaches

Only the construction of a phylogeny does not support its reliability. The confidence of a given phylogenetic hypothesis is assured by support values that can be obtained by different statistical approaches. Some of these approaches are bootstrap, jackknife, Bremer support, and posterior probability. Below, I will argue each of them.

2.4.1. Bootstrap and jackknife

The most popular estimate to test the robustness of a phylogenetic hypothesis is a nonparametric method applied to a phylogenetic analysis by Joseph Felsenstein (1942-) in 1985 [39]. The method comprises a resampling with replenishment of the database. From it, pseudo-alignments (with the same length) are generated from where pseudo-trees will be created.

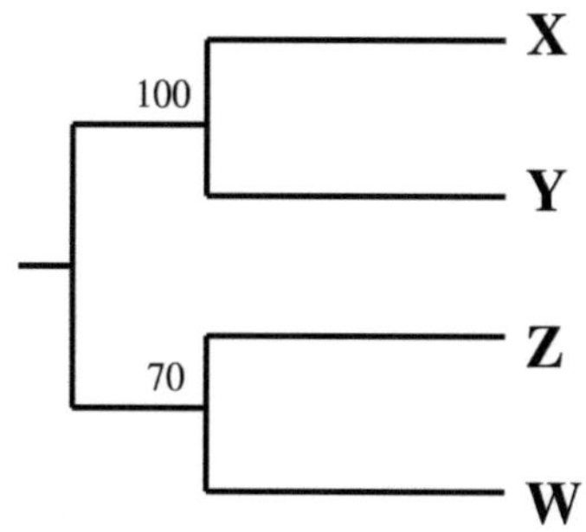

Figure 7. Phylogeny exemplifies how the bootstrap values are exposed on the nodes of the consensus tree. The groups X and Y were together during 100% of the pseudo-trees, whereas Z and W formed a clade in only 70% of them.

The number of replicates will imply the number of pseudo-alignments and generated pseudo-trees [39, 40]. For example, if the number of replicas chosen is 100, then at the end of the analysis we will have 100 pseudo-trees, which can be represented in a single phylogeny and a consensus tree. **Figure 7** shows an example of phylogeny using bootstrap.

The values on the nodes are the bootstrap which is the number of times a given clade has been repeated in pseudo-trees. Controversial groups usually present inconsistencies with low bootstrap values (i.e., below 70%), while consistent groupings present high bootstrap values (close to 100%). The method is used in some phylogenetic inferences as maximum parsimony, neighbor joining, maximum evolution, UPGMA, and maximum likelihood.

Hedges [41] suggests that 2000 replicates increase the accuracy of phylogeny because the p-value bootstrap reaches about ±1% at a 95% confidence limit. Therefore, more than 2000 replicates have little effect and increase the computational time of the analyses.

Jackknife is similar to the bootstrap, but it is an unsampled resampling with subsets of data smaller than the original. In this way, it is possible to know if the exclusion of certain characteristics will have an effect on the topology. It can also be used in analyses of maximum parsimony. For both bootstrap and jackknife, the increase of replicas reduces the standard deviation. For Müller [42] a number of replicates greater than 3458 are unnecessary since it no longer reduces the standard deviation in both confidence estimates.

2.4.2. *Bremer support*

Like previous methods, this method also causes disorders that may reveal data fragility and homoplasies. The support of Bremer also called decay index, however, allows verifying the number of extra steps needed to break a branch in relation to the fewer parsimony trees [43]. It is an important test to test the stability of phylogenies based on parsimony but was originally used in distance analysis [44]. It corresponds to the ratio of the consistency index to the number of steps in a given tree. For example, if the most parsimonious phylogeny has 88 steps, the consistency index will be equal to 1. If another phylogeny based on the same database presents 100 steps, then its consistency index will be 88/100, that is, 0.88 [45]. The method is a good alternative to test the monophyly of taxa whose data were generated by morphological data.

2.4.3. *Posterior probability*

The support value used in Bayesian inference is the posterior probability. It is a way of check the probability of a particular phylogeny, where the probability of the tree is given by P(T), given the data D, or P (T | D). A tree is characterized by the topology τ and associated with the length of β branches. Thus the value of posterior probability is given by [46].

$$\mathbf{P}(\tau \mid \mathbf{D}). \tag{7}$$

The relationship between posterior probability value and bootstrap was not established; however, what is possible to observe is that the same phylogenetic hypothesis presents higher values of posterior probability value than bootstrap [46].

2.5. Phylogenetics software

With the development of different phylogenetic methods and technological advancement, various programs or packages were built. These programs allow the analysis of thousands of data that would be impossible to work manually. Generally, each of the programs for phylogenetic analysis uses different formats of input files. The formats can be of different types, fasta, meg, nexus, phylip, clustal, and MFS format. These formats are generated during the alignment of sequences that can be performed in the programs Clustal X, Clustal W [47], Bioedit [48], and Aliview [49]. Once the alignment is properly formatted, you can then run the analyses in the desired program. In this session, I will present some programs of phylogenetic analysis and general characteristics of them.

2.5.1. *FastTree*

The software is an open source and can be installed on different platforms (Mac, Linux/Unix, and Windows). It has the purpose of doing ML analyses of thousands of DNA, RNA, and protein data much faster than other programs (about 100–1000 times faster). For DNA analysis you can use the Jukes-Cantor and GTR replacement models, which is a limitation. For protein data, it uses the Jones-Taylor-Thornton 1992 (JTT) [50], Whelan and Goldman 2001 (WAG) [51], and Le and Gascuel 2008 (LG) [52] models. One of the great advantages of the program is to use a category of each site (or CAT model) approach, and it reduces the computational time during the analyses, mainly of amino acids [53–55]. The program uses a specific type of support value, called local-bootstrap support values that can vary throughout the search, but the traditional bootstrap can be obtained by using the SEQBOOT program (belonging to the phylogeny inference package) that resamples the data. The program written in Perl CompareToBootstrap.pl. can be used to compare the tree generated by FastTree and this, with resampling of the data. The program uses the multiple sequence alignment (MSA), fasta, and interleaved phylip format formats.

2.5.2. *Molecular evolutionary genetics analysis (MEGA)*

It presents a very friendly graphical interface, besides being free [56, 57]. It also works on Mac, Linux/Unix, and Windows. It has some advantages, such as the ability to perform sequence

http://dx.doi.org/10.5772/intechopen.79422

alignment in the program itself through MUSCLE or Clustal. The program also has the option of looking for the appropriate replacement model for the data (however it is little used for this) and the possibility of constructing the distance matrix. Phylogenies can be based on ML, NJ, minimal evolution, and UPGMA. Bootstrap values can be added to trees or the tree consensus easily by choosing the number of replicas. It allows the analysis of DNA, RNA, and protein and also the distance of the matrix. The tree created can be viewed and edited in the program itself, which increases its practicality than other phylogenetic analysis programs. ML analyses have Jukes-Cartor models, Kimura 2-parameters, Tamura 3-parameters, Hasegawa-Kishino-Yano, and GTR for nucleotide data and 13 models for amino acid sequences (Poisson, equal entry, Dayhoff, JTT, JTT + F, WAG, WAG + F, LG, F + LG, mtREV, mtREV + F, cpREV, cpREV). The version for the Microsoft Windows operating system can execute strings of different extensions (.an, .nexus, .phylip, .gcg, fasta, .pir, .nbrf, .msf, .ig, and .xml) which must be converted into extension. meg, usually found by the program.

2.5.3. MrBayes

It is a most commonly used Bayesian analysis programs [58, 59]. It is also free and serves all major operating systems, but it needs to be compiled in the Unix/Linux version. It allows the analysis of DNA, RNA, and protein restriction sites morphological data and also from a mixed file containing the mixture of these data. The input file is the nexus format. This file, in addition to the nucleotide sequence, protein, etc., should also have additional information such as the specific evolution model and other useful parameters to perform the analysis. The choice of each of the parameters of the input file should be placed with great care, preferably following the steps in the program manual, as errors may interfere with the final result of the analysis.

2.5.4. Phylogenetic analysis using PAUP (PAUP*)

PAUP is one of the most popular software for maximum parsimony, but can also be used in the phylogenetic reconstruction of neighbor-joining. The original version was paid for. Some changes are happening in PAUP version 4.0 of the software; there are options to run on Mac OS X, Windows, and Linux. An open-source command-line version (need the Fortran runtime) is under construction, as is a graphical user interface (GUI) for Windows [60, 61]. According to the developers of the program, the trial versions are still free, but those with a graphical interface will expire, except for the command-line version. The default input file is nexus (.nex). The default input file is nexus (.nex), and all information about the sequence must be in it, such as alignment, substitution model, if the given ones are partitioned and how, if the used sequence is coding, etc. Due to a large amount of data contained in this file, it should be built with care and attention (especially to the symbols accepted by the program), otherwise, a series of bugs will appear. The program is easy to execute, mainly in the version with a graphics interface. It works with DNA, RNA, proteins, and discrete character data (1/0).

2.5.5. Phylogeny inference package (PHYLIP)

It is a package consisting of about 30 programs in C source code. It is free and can be used on Mac, Linux/Unix, and Windows. It has programs that run analysis of parsimony, neighbor Joining, UPGMA, and likelihood. It can create phylogenies based on a distance matrix (fitch program). It is quite versatile working with data from DNA, RNA, amino acid, gene frequency, and discrete character data (1/0). It can use bootstrap or jackknife (SEQBOOT) to determine the support of the branches and also presents a specific program (consense) for building a consensus tree [62–64]. The program does not have a graphics interface and presents few substitution models for both DNA and proteins. However, it performed a large number of phylogenetic methods.

2.5.6. PHYML

The great advantage of the software is to present a likelihood analysis for nucleotides and proteins. Unlike most programs, they only analyze nucleotides. The input file is in phylip (.phy) format. The program is free code and can be installed on all platforms; however, the installation presents particularities that must be respected. It has a list of choices which facilitates its execution and is one of the software with bigger options for models of substitution (JC69, K80, F81, F84, HKY85, etc.). The number of bootstrap replicas is not automatically generated, it must be chosen, with 100 being the default amount. With each replicate, a phylogeny is generated [65–67]. The program currently has smart model selection in PHYML (SMS) [67], another program that assists in the search for the best replacement model for nucleotides and proteins. Both PHYML and SMS have versions for online execution. Although quite versatile, developers recommend that the database has between 100 and 200 sequences and a maximum of 2000 characters. The software becomes slow and consumes a lot of memory with larger banks [67].

2.5.7. Randomized accelerated maximum likelihood (RAXML)

The program is an open source for ML analysis, an alternative to PHYML for long databases. It is derived from dnaml, one of the programs available in PHYLIP [63]. The input files are in phylip (.phy) or fasta (.fas) formats. It can perform binary, nucleotide, and protein data. It is one of the programs that have more options of substitution models for phylogenetic inferences based on data of proteins. It is available for all platforms, but the form of installation depends on the type of platform and also the configuration of the processor. The AVX version can run on more modern processors (e.g., the Intel i7 series or AMD Bulldozer systems) and runs faster than the SSE3 version. In addition, Mac and Linux will have different compilation forms that must meet the instructions in the manual for the correct installation. The likelihood value is more similar to the PHYML values found because they use similar methods, but it is not comparable to those obtained by other ML analysis programs. CAT model of rate heterogeneity can be used in long databases (over 50 taxa) to accelerate the phylogenetic inferences of the initial trees. Later the search of the trees is refined with the use of RΓ (refinement under Γ) search algorithm [68–70].

2.6. Visualization tree tools

Many of the software for phylogenetic construction at the end of the analysis generate a tree in non-graphical, difficult-to-interpret formats. Except for the MEGA program that automatically opens a tree after its construction, most phylogenies will need to be shown using other features, such as Archeopteryx, TreeView, and iTol.

2.6.1. *Archaeopteryx*

It is a free code software that allows viewing and editing of phylogeny. The program is written in Java and this allows it to be installed on all platforms. It can read phylogenies in different formats (phyloXML, newick, nexus, nhx, etc.). The options are quite versatile, being possible to edit different informations (color, root, form of phylogeny, etc.) [71–77]. It is important that the user fully exploits the program and chooses the best options to represent their phylogeny.

2.6.2. *Dendroscope*

The software is written in Java available for all platforms. It is an easy-to-use program, but it does not have editing options as sophisticated as Archeopteryx. It accepts the formats nexml, .dendro, .tre, and nexus and also has different options for editing phylogenies [71, 72].

2.6.3. *iTol*

It can be used online and has several editing possibilities. Phylogenies can be seen in a circular, normal, or non-root fashion. Branches can be colored differently for better identification of taxonomic groups. The program also allows the addition of captions, connections, heat maps, box plots, protein domains, and annotation data. The input files can be of the newick, nexus, phyloXML, jplance, QIIMe2, and NHX types [73, 74].

2.6.4. *TreeView*

The open-source software can interpret a large number of phylogeny formats [75, 76]. It is quite simple and easy to use, but it does not have editing options as sophisticated as Archeopteryx.

2.7. Gene tree versus species tree

Not all phylogenetic reconstructions can reflect the evolutionary history of a group; sometimes the evolutionary history of the gene is shown in the phylogenetic hypothesis. Pamilo and Nei [77] emphasized that it is important to distinguish between a gene tree and species tree. Gene tree shows the history of paralogous genes in different species. While the specie tree reflects the processes of speciation within a lineage, through the use of orthologous genes. Orthologs have similar functions among the organisms that possess them.

The genes undergo multiple duplication processes and may present multiple copies with distinct functions in the genome of the same species, as an example, the glycosyltransferase 6 gene family, which possesses the ABO gene. Some parallel copies may still lose function in some groups and become pseudogenes, as an example GGTA1 in Catarrhini (human, apes, and old world monkeys) [78]. **Figure 8** shows the difference between two types of homologous genes.

The misuse of paralogous genes while attempting to construct the phylogeny of a taxon is a recurring problem and needs the care to ensure the use of orthologous genes. The most effective procedure is to verify the similarity of the target sequence through the basic local

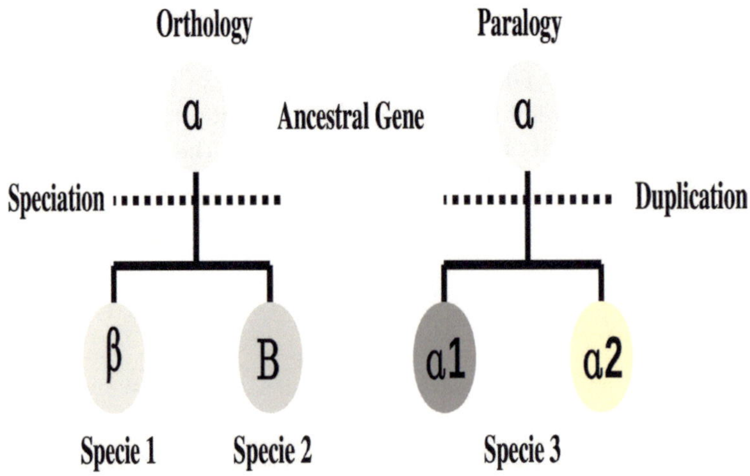

Figure 8. Difference between orthologous genes and paralogs, when the ancestral gene is being represented by α. The first phylogenetic tree shows the origin of the orthologues β and B, coming from the speciation between species 1 and 2. The second phylogeny represents the process of formation by duplication of the genes α1 and α2.

alignment search tool (BLAST) and to analyze the results with the best scores (with the lowest values of e-value). The orthologous gene will tend to exhibit more similarities than the paralogs (one of the parallel graphic copies maintains the original function, while others may have multiple mutations). Another strategy is to verify in the literature whether the target gene has copies within the genome of the species analyzed.

The third type of homologous gene may compromise the validity of a phylogenetic hypothesis, the xenologous genes, which were obtained by horizontal event gene transfer (HGT) between two species. Although they may act as phylogenetic artifacts, these genes are of extremely evolutionary importance (the possibility of contamination should be considered first). They can be easily identified through the BLAST tool, which shows rather unusual results, indicating similarities between the target sequence and others of bacterial or viral origin. These genes are quite common among prokaryotes, and the best known are those related to antibiotic resistance. HGT also played a key role in the evolution of eukaryotes, mainly in the origin of this domain from several events of serial endosymbiosis, fundamental in the acquisition of nucleus and organelles [79]. Another striking example was the syncytin gene, originated from reiterated endogenous retrovirus (ERV) sequences that were fundamental in the formation of placental structures in eutherian mammals [80, 81].

2.8. Tree of life

From Charles Darwin to today, it is difficult to determine what would be the real tree of life, complete and unequivocal. What is concrete today is that life is composed of the domains (or superkingdom) Bacteria, Eukarya, and Archaea [82]. The proposal of the third group was observed by Carl Woese and George Fox based on the 16S ribosomal gene [83]. This taxonomic proposal is shown in **Figure 9**. The relationships between these three groups are controversial. Bacteria has the wall cellular with peptidoglycans, different from members of Archaea and Eukarya.

http://dx.doi.org/10.5772/intechopen.79422

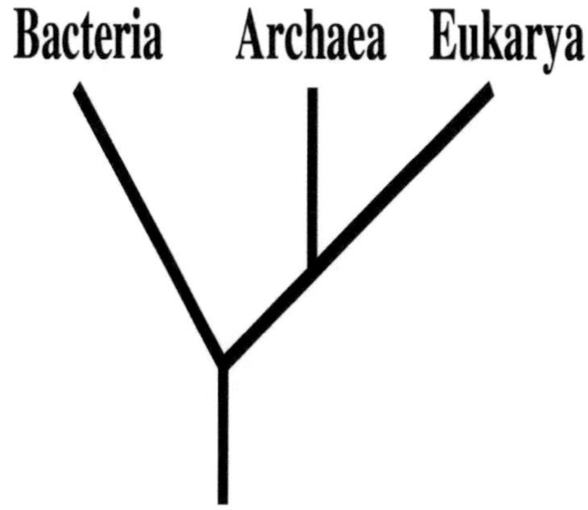

Figure 9. The three domains (or superkingdom) of life: Bacteria, Archaea and Eukarya.

These two groups, in turn, have similar replication, transcription, and translation mechanisms. However, only Eukarya has a cytoskeleton containing tubulin and actin [83, 84]. Thus, although this classification is robust, it still needs more information about a possible LUCA.

3. Conclusions

Phylogenetic systematics emphasized the investigation of phylogenetic relationships among living beings. However, this view is pre-Darwinian and had supporters over 2 millennia ago, in antique Greece. From then on, the relationships of ancestry between living beings are described as cladograms constructed from homologies and homoplasies. The computational advancement allowed new methods and phylogenetic approaches based on advanced mathematical assumptions. As a result, current free computational tools are rising, aiming at the analysis of long databases faster and higher, and with fewer phylogenetic artifacts (such as homoplasies). Each method and software, however, should be appropriate to the database (sample number and a number of characters) and computational power. But deserves attention in terms of the support value that differs from that applied in classical methods. Visualization and editing of phylogenies are further possible through various tools easy to install and run. Despite all the advantages, it is essential that the researcher knows what evolutionary history wants to produce in his phylogeny, whether it is the genes or species history. For this, it is indispensable to identify orthologous, paralogues, and xenologous genes. It is frequent for concatenated analysis of these genes to generate a puzzling and unclear phylogeny. It is important to consider that each gene can show ancestral histories of particular lineages, such as 16S gene which provided the tree of life, comprising the Bacteria, Eukarya, and Archaea domains.

Conflict of interest

The author has declared that no competing interests exist.

Author details

Eliane Barbosa Evanovich dos Santos

Address all correspondence to: lianevanovich@gmail.com

Laboratório de Genética Humana e Médica, Instituto de Ciências Biológicas—Universidade Federal do Pará, Pará, Brasil

References

[1] Pallas PS. Elenchus zoophytorum sistens generum adumbrationes generaliores et specierum cognitarum succintas descriptiones, cum selectis auctorum synonymis. The Hague (The Netherlands): Apud Petrum van Cleef, 1766

[2] Trevisanato SI. Reconstructing anaximander's biological model unveils a theory of evolution akin to darwin's, though centuries before the birth of science. Acta Medico-Historica Adriatica. 2016;**14**:63-72

[3] Couprie DL, Kočandrle R. Anaximander's 'Boundless Nature'. Peitho examina. antiqua. 2013;**1**:63-91

[4] Dunn PM. Aristotle (384-322 bc): philosopher and scientist of ancient Greece. Archives of Disease in Childhood. Fetal and Neonatal Edition. 2006;**91**:F75-F77

[5] Ragan MA. Trees and networks before and after Darwin. Biology Direct. 2009;**4**(43)

[6] von Lieven AF, Humar M. A Cladistic Analysis of Aristotle's Animal Groups in the Historia animalium. History and Philosophy of the Life Sciences. 2008;**30**:227-262

[7] Müller-Wille S, Charmantier I. Natural history and information overload: The case of Linnaeus. Studies in History and Philosophy of Science Part C: Studies in History and Philosophy of Biological and Biomedical Sciences. 2012;**43**:4-15

[8] Paterlini M. There shall be order. The legacy of Linnaeus in the age of molecular biology. EMBO Reports. 2007;**8**:814-816

[9] Darwin C. On the origin of species. London: Murray; 1859

[10] Phylogenetic Systematics HW. Annual Review of Entomology. 1965;**10**:97-116

[11] Andersen NM. The impact of W. Hennig's "phylogenetic systematics" on contemporary entomology. European Journal of Entomology. 2001;**98**:133-150

[12] Jensen RJ. Phenetics: revolution, reform or natural consequence? Taxon. 2009;**58**:50-60

[13] Brooks, DR, Caira JN, Platt TR, Pritchard MH. Principles and methods of phylogenetic systematics : a cladistics workbook. 1984. Harvard Botany Libraries. University of Kansas, Lawrence, USA

[14] Dupuis C. Willi Hennig's impact on taxonomic thought. Annual Review of Ecology and Systematics. 1984;**15**:1-25

[15] Mount DW. Maximum Parsimony Method for Phylogenetic Prediction. CSH Protocols. 2008;**3**

[16] Bergsten J. A review of long-branch attraction. Cladistics. 2005;**21**:163-193

[17] Gregor I, Steinbrück L, McHardy AC. PTree: pattern-based, stochastic search for maximum parsimony phylogenies. Peer-reviewed Journal. 2013;**25**:e89

[18] Hoang DT, Vinh LS, Flouri T, Stamatakis A, von Haeseler A, Minh BQ. MPBoot: fast phylogenetic maximum parsimony tree inference and bootstrap approximation. BMC Evolutionary Biology. 2018 Feb 2;**18**(1):11

[19] Hoang DT, Chernomor O, von Haeseler A, Minh BQ, Vinh LS. UFBoot2: Improving the Ultrafast Bootstrap Approximation. Molecular Biology and Evolution. 2018;**35**:518-522

[20] Saitou N, Nei M. The neighbor-joining method: a new method for reconstructing phylogenetic trees. Molecular Biology and Evolution. 1987;**4**:406-425

[21] Nascimento M, Sousa A, Ramirez M, Francisco AP, Carriço JA, Vaz C. PHYLOViZ 2.0: providing scalable data integration and visualization for multiple phylogenetic inference methods. Bioinformatics. 2017;**33**:128-129

[22] Hedge J, Wilson DJ. Bacterial Phylogenetic Reconstruction from Whole Genomes Is Robust to Recombination but Demographic Inference Is Not. MBio Journal. 2014;**5**:e02158-e02114

[23] Cavalli-Sforza LL, Edwards AW. Phylogenetic analysis. Models and estimation procedures. American Journal of Human Genetics. 1967;**19**:233-257

[24] Cho A. Constructing Phylogenetic Trees Using Maximum Likelihood. Scripps Senior Theses. 2012;**46**

[25] Posada D, Crandall KAMODELTEST. testing the model of DNA substitution. Bioinformatics. 1998;**14**:817-818

[26] Darriba D, Taboada GL, Doallo R, Posada D. jModelTest 2: more models. new heuristics and parallel computing. Nature Methods. 2012;**772**

[27] Gaut BS, Lewis PO. Success of maximum-likelihood phylogeny inference in the 4-taxon case. Molecular Biology and Evolution. 1995;**12**:152-162

[28] Huelsenbeck JP. Performance of phylogenetic methods insimulation. Systematic Biology. 1995;**44**:17-48

[29] Chang JT. Inconsistency of evolutionary tree topology reconstruction methods when substitution rates vary across char-acters. Mathematical Biosciences. 1996;**134**:189-215

[30] Lockhart PJ, Larkum AWD, Steel MA, Waddell PJ, Penny D. Evolution of chlorophyll and bacteriochlorophyll: theproblem of invariant sites in sequence analysis. PNAS. 1996;**93**:1930-1934

[31] Cavalli-Sforza LL, Edwards AWF. Phylogenetic analysis: models and estimation procedures. Evolution. 1967;**21**:550-570

[32] Yang Z, Rannala B. Bayesian phylogenetic inference using DNA sequences: a Markov Chain Monte Carlo Method. Molecular Biology and Evolution. 1997;**14**:717-724

[33] Rannala B, Yang Z. Probability distribution of molecular evolutionary trees: a new method of phylogenetic inference. Journal of Molecular Evolution. 1996;**43**:304-311

[34] Nascimento F, Reis M. Yang Z. A biologist's guide to Bayesian phylogenetic analysis. Nature Ecology & Evolution. 2017;**1**:1446-1454

[35] Suzuki Y, Glazko GV, Nei M. Overcredibility of molecular phylogenies obtained by Bayesian phylogenetics. PNAS. 2002;**99**:16138-16143

[36] Alfaro ME, Zoller S. Lutzoni f. Bayes or bootstrap? A simulation study comparing the performance of Bayesian Markov chain Monte Carlo sampling and bootstrapping in assessing phylogenetic confidence. Molecular Biology and Evolution. 2003;**20**:255-266

[37] Douady CJ. Delsuc f, Boucher Y, Doolittle WF, Douzery EJP. Comparison of Bayesian and maximum likelihood bootstrap measures of phylogenetic reliability. Molecular Biology and Evolution. 2003;**20**:248-254

[38] Lewis PO, Holder MT, Polytomies HKE. Bayesian phylogenetic inference. Systematic Biology. 2005;**54**:241-253

[39] Felsenstein J. Confidence Limits on Phylogenies: An Approach Using the Bootstrap. Evolution. 1985;**39**:783-791

[40] Efron B, Halloran E, Holmes S. Bootstrap confidence levels for phylogenetic trees. PNAS. 1996;**93**:7085-7090

[41] Hedges SB. The number of replications needed for accurate estimation of the bootstrap P value in phylogenetic studies. Molecular Biology and Evolution. 1992;**9**:366-369

[42] Müller KF. The efficiency of different search strategies in estimating parsimony jackknife, bootstrap. and Bremer support. BMC Evolutionary Biology. 2005;**5**:58

[43] Bremer K. Branch support and tree stability. Cladistics. 1994;**10**:295-304

[44] Farris JS, Kluge AG, Mickevich MF. Immunological Distance and the Phylogenetic Relationships of the Rana boylii Species Group. Systematic Zoology. 1982;**31**:479-491

[45] Bremer K. The limits of amino acid sequence data in angiosperm phylogenetic recontruction. Evolution. 1988;**42**:795-803

[46] Cummings MP, Handley SA, Myers DS, Reed DL, Rokas A, Winka K. Comparing bootstrap and posterior probability values in the four-taxon case. Systematic Biology. 2003;**52**:477-487

[47] Larkin MA1, Blackshields G, Brown NP, Chenna R, McGettigan PA, McWilliam H, Valentin F, Wallace IM, Wilm A, Lopez R, Thompson JD, Gibson TJ, Higgins DG. Clustal W and Clustal X version 2.0. Bioinformatics. 2007;**23**:2947-2948

[48] Hall TA. Bioedit: a user-friendly biological sequence aligniment editor and analysis program for windows 95/98/NT. Nucleic acids symposium series. 1999:95-98

[49] Larsson AAV. a fast and lightweight alignment viewer and editor for large data sets. Bioinformatics. 2014;**30**:3276-3278

[50] Jones DT, Taylor WR, Thornton JM. The rapid generation of mutation data matrices from protein sequences. Computer Applications in the Biosciences. 1992;**8**:275-282

[51] Whelan S. Goldman N. A general empirical model of protein evolution derived from multiple protein families using a maximum-likelihood approach. Molecular Biology and Evolution. 2001;**18**:691-699

[52] Le SQ, Gascuel O. An improved general amino acid replacement matrix. Molecular Biology and Evolution. 2008;**25**:1307-1320

[53] Le SQ, Lartillot N, Gascuel O. Phylogenetic mixture models for proteins. Philosophical Transactions of the Royal Society of London. Series B, Biological Sciences. 2008;**363**: 3965-3976

[54] Price MN, Dehal PS, Arkin APFT. Computing Large Minimum-Evolution Trees with Profiles instead of a Distance Matrix. Molecular Biology and Evolution. 2009;**26**:1641-1650. DOI: 10.1093/molbev/msp077

[55] FastTree [Internet]. 2018. Available from: http://www.microbesonline.org/fasttree/ [Accessed: 2018-06-06]

[56] Kumar S, Stecher G, Tamura K. MEGA7: Molecular evolutionary genetics analysis version 7.0 for bigger datasets. Molecular Biology and Evolution. 2016;**33**:1870-1874

[57] MEGA [Internet]. 2018. Available from: https://www.megasoftware.net [Accessed: 2018-06-06]

[58] Ronquist F, Huelsenbeck JPMRBAYES. 3: Bayesian phylogenetic inference under mixed models. Bioinformatics. 2003;**19**:1572-1574

[59] MrBayes [Internet]. 2018. Available from: http://mrbayes.sourceforge.net/manual.php [Accessed: 2018-06-06]

[60] Maddison DR, Swofford DL, Maddison WPNEXUS. an extensible file format for systematic information. Systematic biology. 2003;**46**:590-621

[61] PAUP* [Internet]. 2018. Available from: https://paup.phylosolutions.com [Accessed: 2018-06-06]

[62] Felsenstein J. PHYLIP (Phylogeny Inference Package) version 3.7a. Distributed by the Author. Department of Genome Sciences, University of Washington, Seattle. 2009

[63] PHYLIP [Internet]. 2018. Available from: http://evolution.genetics.washington.edu/phylip/getme-new1.html [Accessed: Jun 6, 2018]

[64] Felsenstein J. PHYLIP—Phylogeny Inference Package (Version 3.2). Cladistics. 1989;**5**: 164-166

[65] Guindon S, Gascuel O. PhyML: A simple, fast and accurate algorithm to estimate large phylogenies by maximum likelihood. Systematic Biology. 2003;**52**:696-704

[66] PHYML [Internet]. 2018. Available from: http://www.atgc-montpellier.fr/phyml/ [Accessed: 2018-06-06]

[67] Lefort V, Longueville JE, Gascuel OSMS. Smart Model Selection in PhyML. Molecular Biology and Evolution. 2017;**34**:2422-2424

[68] Stamatakis A. RAxML Version 8: A tool for Phylogenetic Analysis and Post-Analysis of Large Phylogenies. Bioinformatics. 2014;**30**:1312-1313

[69] RAXML [Internet]. 2018. Available from: https://sco.h-its.org/exelixis/web/software/raxml/index.html [Accessed: 2018-06-06]

[70] RAXML [Internet]. 2018. Available from: https://sco.h-its.org/exelixis/web/software/raxml/index.html [Accessed: Jun 6, 2018]

[71] Huson DH, Scornavacca C. Dendroscope 3: An interactive tool for rooted phylogenetic-trees and networks. Systematic Biology. 2012;**61**:1061-1067

[72] Dendroscope 3 [Internet]. 2018. Available from: http://dendroscope.org [Accessed: Jun 6, 2018]

[73] Ciccarelli FD, Doerks T, von Mering C, Creevey CJ, Snel B, Bork P. Toward automatic reconstruction of a highly resolved tree of life. Science 2006;**311**:1283-1287

[74] iTol [Internet]. 2018. Available from: https://sco.h-its.org/exelixis/web/software/raxml/index. html [Accessed: Jun 6, 2018]

[75] Page RDMTREEVIEW. An application to display phylogenetic trees on personal computers. Computer Applications in the Biosciences. 1996;**12**:357-358

[76] Treeview [Internet]. 2018. Available from: http://taxonomy.zoology.gla.ac.uk/rod/treeview.html [Accessed: Jun 6, 2018]

[77] Pamilo P, Nei M. Relationships between Gene Trees and Species Trees. Molecular Biology and Evolution. 1988;**5**:568-583

[78] Galili U. Significance of the Evolutionary α1,3-galactosyltransferase (GGTA1) gene inactivation in preventing extinction of apes and old world monkeys. Journal of Molecular Evolution. 2015;**80**:1-9

[79] Keeling PJ, Palmer JD. Horizontal gene transfer in eukaryotic evolution. Nature Reviews Genetics. 2008;**9**:605-618

[80] Cornelis G, Heidmann O, Degrelle SA, Vernochet C, Lavialle C, Letzelter C, et al. Captured retroviral envelope syncytin gene associated with the unique placental structure of higher ruminants. PNAS. 2013;**110**:E828-E837

[81] Lavialle C, Cornelis G, Dupressoir A, Esnault C, Heidmann O, Vernochet C. Heidmann T Paleovirology of 'syncytins', retroviral env genes exapted for a role in placentation. Philosophical Transactions. 2013;**368**:20120507

[82] Woese CR, Kandler O, Wheelis ML. Towards a natural system of organisms: Proposal for the domains Archaea, Bacteria, and Eucarya. PNAS. 1990;**87**:4576-4579

[83] Woese CR, Fox GE. Phylogenetic structure of the prokaryotic domain: The primary kingdoms. PNAS. 1977;**74**:5088-5090

[84] Doolittle WF. Phylogenetic classification and the universal tree. Science. 1999;**284**: 2124-2129

Chapter 2

Phylogeny of Three Palmwine Yeasts Genera

Ogueri Nwaiwu

Additional information is available at the end of the chapter

http://dx.doi.org/10.5772/intechopen.79958

Abstract

Sequences from three palm wine yeast genera namely *Saccharomyces cerevisiae, Pichia kudriavzevii,* and *Candida ethanolica* were analyzed to establish their phylogenetic relationships, geographical origin, and food matrix source of their close relatives. Up to 600 sequences present in yeasts representing close relatives of palm wine yeasts were examined. Pyhlogenetic trees constructed showed polyphyletic relationships in *C. ethanolica* whereas close relatives of *S. cerevisiae* and *P. kudriavzevii* showed little divergence. Sequence data for both *Elaeis* sp. and *Raphia* sp. palm trees showed that highest number of palm wine yeasts relatives sequence submissions to the Genbank were from China and beverages were mainly the sources of close relatives of *S. cerevisiae* and *P. kudriavzevii* whereas *C. ethanolica* closest relatives were from various non-food sources. Overall relatives of palm wine yeasts were not specific to any particular food or fermentation mix. The guanine-cytosine (G+C) content in *P. kudriavzevii* (57–58%) and *C. ethanolica* (56–57%) was higher than that of *S. cerevisiae* (47.3–51%). This suggests that the *P. kudriavzevii* and *C. ethanolica* have a higher recombination rate than *S. cerevisiae* strains analyzed. The data may help to understand palm wine yeast conservation and the diverse food matrixes and geographical origins where their close relatives exist.

Keywords: yeasts, phylogeny, *Saccharomyces cerevisiae, Pichia kudriavzevii, Candida ethanolica*

1. Introduction

Palm wine is a traditional drink consumed mainly in sub-Saharan Africa, parts of Asia, and South America. It is obtained from fermentation of saps of different palm trees. Palm wine is sourced from palm trees and they grow throughout tropical and subtropical regions with just a few species found in temperate regions possibly due to freeze intolerance of seedlings [1]. The method of obtaining the drink by tapping has been described in many reports [2] and the

IntechOpen

© 2018 The Author(s). Licensee IntechOpen. This chapter is distributed under the terms of the Creative Commons Attribution License (http://creativecommons.org/licenses/by/3.0), which permits unrestricted use, distribution, and reproduction in any medium, provided the original work is properly cited. CC BY

palm sap varies according to palm trees found in different geographical location. Yeasts are the main organisms implicated in the fermentation of the drink and they exist as natural flora on palm trees. Irrespective of the palm tree source, a common feature of the drink is that it goes sour within 24 h unless it is subjected to cold storage. The two trees from which palm wine is mostly tapped in Nigeria are *Raphia hookeri* and *Elaeis guineensis*. There is a debate on the possible origin or source of these palm trees. The tree *Raphia hookeri* is known as the wine palm and is the most widespread familiar Raphia palm in fresh water swamps of west and central Africa [3]. Many local varieties exist in the tropical rain forest of Nigeria and it is also grown in India, Malaysia, and Singapore [4]. The *E. guineensis* oil palm variety is more widely found around the world. A report pointed out that *E. guineensis* palm tree originated in the tropical rain forest region of West Africa and can be found in Cameroon, Côte d'Ivoire, Ghana, Liberia, Nigeria, Sierra Leone, Togo Angola, and the Congo [5]. It is believed in the report that during the fourteenth to seventeenth centuries, some palm fruits were taken to the Americas and from there to the Far East where it thrived. Yeast are known to reflect human history [6] hence it is possible the yeast strains found in palm wine were introduced to new regions via the plant materials introduced in those locations.

Although it is known that yeasts have been used for food and beverage fermentations [7] hundreds of years ago and domestication is believed to have been initiated before the discovery of microbes [8], the extent of genetic diversity is still under study around the world. Recent reports have shown that non-*Saccharomyces* yeasts have different oenological properties to those of *S. cerevisiae* [9]. Other reports emphasize that even though biochemical and genomic studies of *S. cerevisiae* have helped our understanding of yeasts, the other lesser known yeast species have not been fully exploited [10]. More understanding of *S. cerevisiae* and non-*S. cerevisiae* yeasts in palm wine is needed [11] in order to get more information on the capabilities of yeasts present in the drink or to probe for novel species [12]. To generate more information, molecular characterization has been used by many investigators and this has led to proper identification of new yeast strains in the drink. The diversity of yeasts from palm wine has not had much in-depth investigation and reports that show evolutionary trees which are the basic structures necessary to establish the relationships among organisms [13] are few in literature. This chapter examines evolutionary relationships of palm wine yeasts and their close relatives based on 26S rRNA sequence data and aims to shed more light on the diversity of yeasts found in the drink.

2. Methodology

2.1. Ribosomal ribonucleic acid genes partial sequence data

In a previous study [2], partial 26S rRNA gene sequences from 18 palm wine yeast isolates were deposited under accession numbers (HG452325-42). The sequences from three yeasts genera identified in that study namely *S. cerevisiae, P. kudriavzevii*, and *C. ethanolica* from *Elaeis* sp. and *Raphia* sp. palm trees were selected and used to carry out new updated searches in this report. For *Elaeis* sp., the sequence accession numbers used were HG425336, HG425328, and HG425333 whereas HG425332, HG425338, and HG425335 were used for the *Raphia* sp. palm tree. The current versions of the selected six sequences mentioned above were used separately for an updated search in the Genbank database. The searches were optimized for highly similar sequences and the first 100 sequences from relatives of each yeast species with the highest percent identity were marked to make a shortlist of up to 600 sequences. These sequences were examined for the features listed at the time of submission after which the countries of origin and sources were noted. Sources were classified as beverage, food, or non-food sources.

2.2. Construction of phylogenetic trees

Phylogenetic trees were constructed from the shortlisted sequences by using the molecular evolutionary genetic analysis (MEGA, version 7) computer software [14]. The software allowed a seamless transfer of the sequences from Genbank. Using the multiple sequence comparison by log expectation (MUSCLE) reported by Edgar [15], multiple sequence alignments (MSA) were constructed with the software. The evolutionary history was inferred by using the maximum likelihood method based on the Tamura-Nei model [16]. The tree with the highest log likelihood was chosen. Initial trees for the heuristic search were obtained using the maximum composite likelihood approach. Trees were drawn to scale, with branch lengths measured in the number of substitutions per site. All positions containing gaps and missing data were eliminated. The nucleic acid composition of the sequences was calculated automatically by switching to the nucleic acids estimation mode of the software after which the G+C content of the sequences were calculated manually from the arginine, guanine, cytosine, and thiamine percentage distribution displayed. The MAS tool MUSCLE used assumes an equality of substitution rates among sites and takes into account differences in transitional, transversional rates, and G+C-content bias [17]. For brevity, only 20 sequences from the initial 100 relatives obtained are shown in the trees with the reference sequence.

The complete list of 600 sequences analyzed showing sources and countries of origin is available in the public repository figshare [18].

3. Results and discussion

3.1. Evolutionary relationships of palm wine yeasts and their relatives

Yeasts facilitate several industrial food fermentation processes, which often consist of a desired specific strain [19]. This may be why domestication is believed to be the main driver of specific yeast prevalence in a geographical location. The understanding of the ecological basis of yeast diversity in nature remains fragmented and cross-kingdom competition has been proposed as a method to generate industrially useful yeast strains with new metabolic traits [20]. Palm wine yeasts are yet to enjoy significant diversity study hence a look at their relatives will enable more information to be generated.

In the last decade, there has been increase in submissions of palm wine yeast sequences based on 26S rRNA genes mainly due to quality checks by academic journals. The identification of new strains is accompanied by performing a search with the basic local alignment search tool [21] followed by submission of DNA sequences to the GenBank. According to Benson et al. [22], GenBank is a comprehensive database that contains publicly available nucleotide sequences for up to 370,000 formally described species. It is common knowledge that these submissions which contain a lot of information are generated mainly through submissions from investigators around the world. Each sequence data received is curated by the GenBank annotation staff to ensure that it is free from errors after which accession numbers are assigned.

All the sequences used in this study were the first versions submitted by investigators. The maximum likelihood method was preferred for the trees constructed because it is computationally intense and all possible trees are considered. Also the method can be useful for widely divergent groups or other difficult situations [23].

3.2. *Candida ethanolica*

The yeast *C. ethanolica* is not widely reported in palm wine. It has been reported as a non-conventional yeast which may present massive resource of yeast biodiversity for industrial applications because it has been found to be adapted to some of the stress factors present in harsh environmental [24]. In that report, it was found that *C. ethanolica* tolerated up to 7% v/v ethanol. This could be useful information for new palm wine drink development especially now that there is increasing interest in non-*Saccharomyces* yeasts with peculiar features able to replace or accompany *S. cerevisiae* during specific industrial fermentations [25].

The *C. ethanolica* strain from *Raphia* sp. (**Figure 1**) and *Elaeis* sp. (**Figure 2**) palm wine showed close relationships with other *Candida* species. The relatives of *Raphia* sp. palm wine that emanated from the same node (**Figure 1**) came from diverse sources. The flanking close relatives (KY283163 and DQ466540) of *C. ethanolica* (HG425332) were isolated from composite microbial powders for aquaculture in China [26] and composite cocoa fermentation in Ghana [27]. Other close relatives included species from the genus *Pichia*. The *P. deserticola* strain (KM005182) from the same node as the reference strain was from aerobic deterioration of total mixed ration silage in China [28]. For *Elaeis* sp. (**Figure 2**) palm wine, close relatives to *C. ethanolica* (HG425336) strain were from a laboratory culture collection with unidentified source [29] and a tannin tolerant yeasts associated with naturally fermented *Miang* leaves in Thailand [30]. A close *P. deserticola* strain of unstated source in GenBank was from a large characterization study [31].

In both *Elaeis* sp. and *Raphia* sp. palm wine, several monophyletic groups were formed with other *Pichia* species namely *P. deserticola*, *P. Manshurica* and *P. galeiformis* which indicate polyphyletic relationships. The polyphyletic nature of *Pichia* has been demonstrated by Kurtzman and Robnett [29] in the analysis of gene sequences that included all known ascomycetous yeasts. Apart from possible similar conserved regions, previous nomenclature at the time of submission of the sequences may also be the reason why *Pichia* species of different genus were observed as close relatives of *C. ethanolica* from *Elaeis* sp. and *Raphia* sp. palm trees.

It has been reported that ascomycetic fungi submitted to the database previously have been assigned names based on their life stages [32, 33]. For example, it was shown that the name for the fungi *Candida krusei* is based on the anamorphic stage whereas its telemorph stage

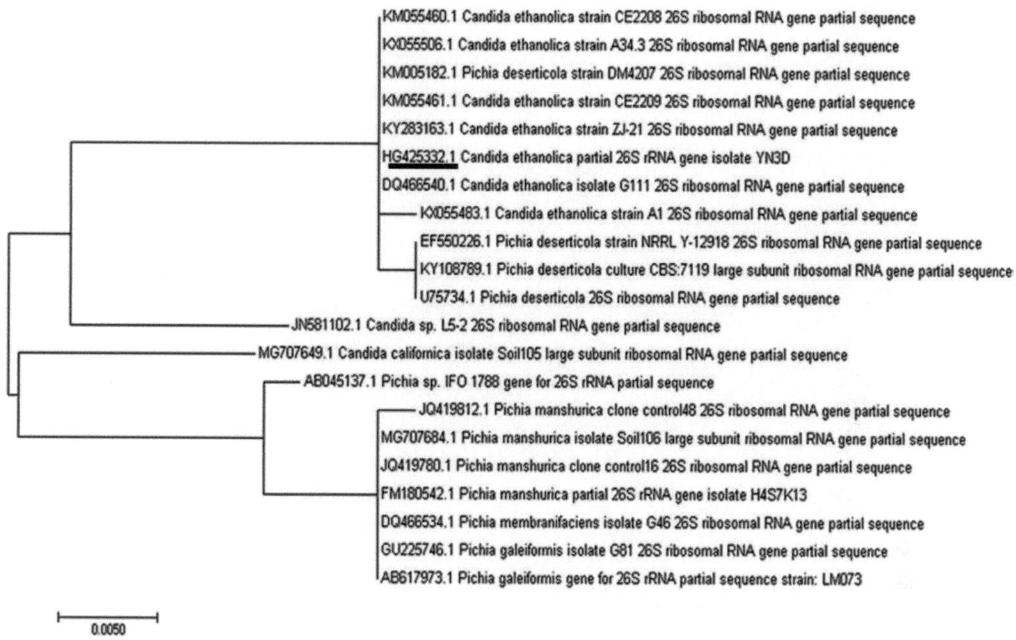

Figure 1. Phylogenetic analysis of *Candida ethanolica* (HG425332-underlined) from *Raphia* sp. palm wine. The tree is drawn to scale, with branch lengths measured in the number of substitutions per site.

name is *Pichia kudriavzevii*. It also has an older name *Issatchenkia orientalis*. The whole *Candida* species consists of up to 850 organisms, which can be distantly related [34]. Hence in order to avoid the confusion, the International Botanical Congress in Melbourne in July 2011, made a change in the international code of nomenclature for fungi and adopted the principle of one fungus can only have one name and ended the system of permitting separate names to be used for anamorphs [35]. The report emphasized that this validated all legitimate names proposed for a species, regardless of what stage they were typed and can serve as the correct name for that species.

3.3. *Sachharomyces cerevisiae*

The yeast *S. cerevisiae* is generally known to be the most used microorganism in the food and drink manufacturing sector. The organism is the dominant yeast species isolated from many studies on palm wine. However, it is unclear whether *S. cerevisiae* as a species occurs naturally or exists solely as a domesticated species [36]. *S. cerevisiae* strains are genetically diverse, largely as a result of human efforts to develop strains specifically adapted to various fermentation processes. These adaptive pressures from various ecological niches may generate behavioral differences among these strains [37]. In a review [8], it was suggested that domestication in *Saccharomyces*, is most pronounced in beer strains, because they live in their industrial niche always and allow only limited genetic admixture with wild stocks and minimal contact with natural environments. Due to this restriction, it was pointed out that

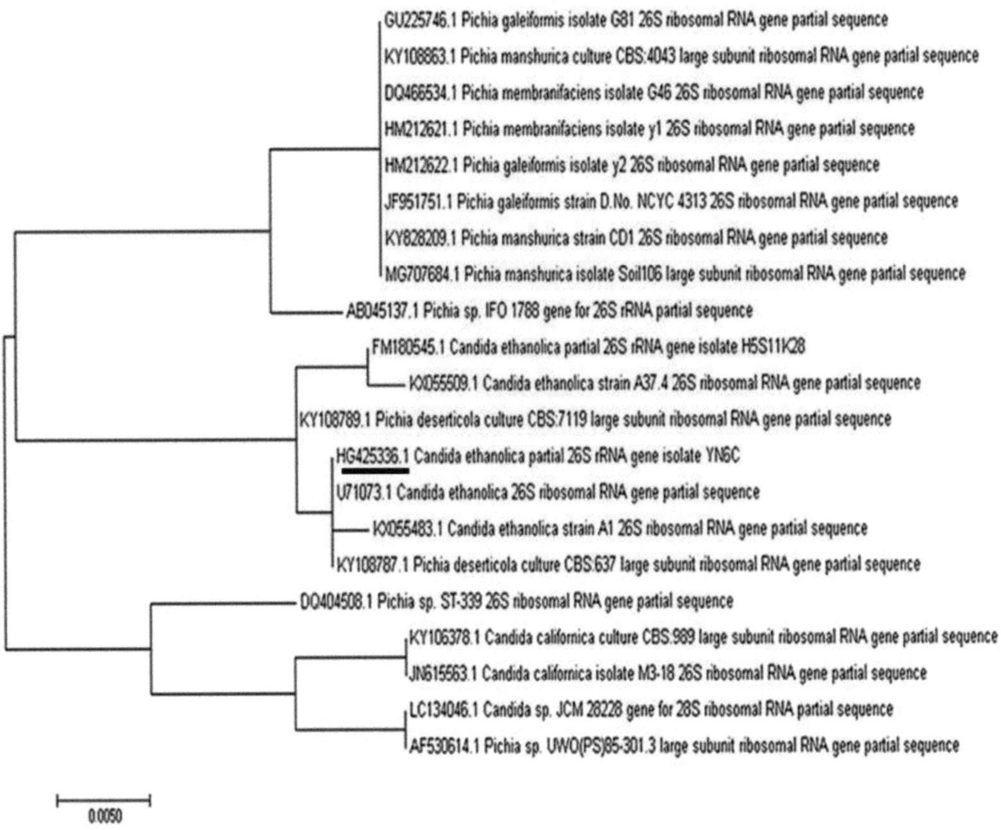

Figure 2. Phylogenetic analysis of *Candida ethanolica* (HG425336-underlined) from *Elaeis* sp. palm wine. The tree is drawn to scale, with branch lengths measured in the number of substitutions per site.

beer yeast genomes show complex patterns of domestication and divergence, making both ale (*S. cerevisiae*) and lager (*S. pastorianus*) strains ideal models to study domestication.

The relatives of palm wine *S. cerevisiae* was not distributed among many species or different genus observed for *Candida species*. Two nodes were observed for the *S. cerevisiae* trees constructed for *Elaeis* sp. (**Figure 3**) and *Raphia* sp. (**Figure 4**). The yeast strain isolated from *Elaeis* sp. (**Figure 3**) was in a different branch from most of its relative whereas it was vice versa for the palm wine yeast from *Raphia* sp. (**Figure 4**) palm wine. As observed for *Candida species*, isolation of *S. cerevisiae* species was from different sources. The close relatives flanking the palm wine strain from *Elaeis* sp. palm wine (HG425328, **Figure 3**) with accession numbers KU862639 and MF966566 were isolated from grape surface [38] and pear sough dough [39] whereas the close relatives of *Raphia* sp. palm wine (HG425338, **Figure 4**) with accession numbers GU080046 and HM191669 were isolated from must of spontaneous fermentation [40] and grape juice used to brew *Musalais*, a beverage made from compressed grapes [41].

It is believed that 99% of yeasts is still unknown [42], and *S. cerevisiae* fermentation could be specific to a particular substrate, hence more studies of *S. cerevisiae* from different palm trees will be beneficial. The genus *Saccharomyces* was previously divided into two groups namely

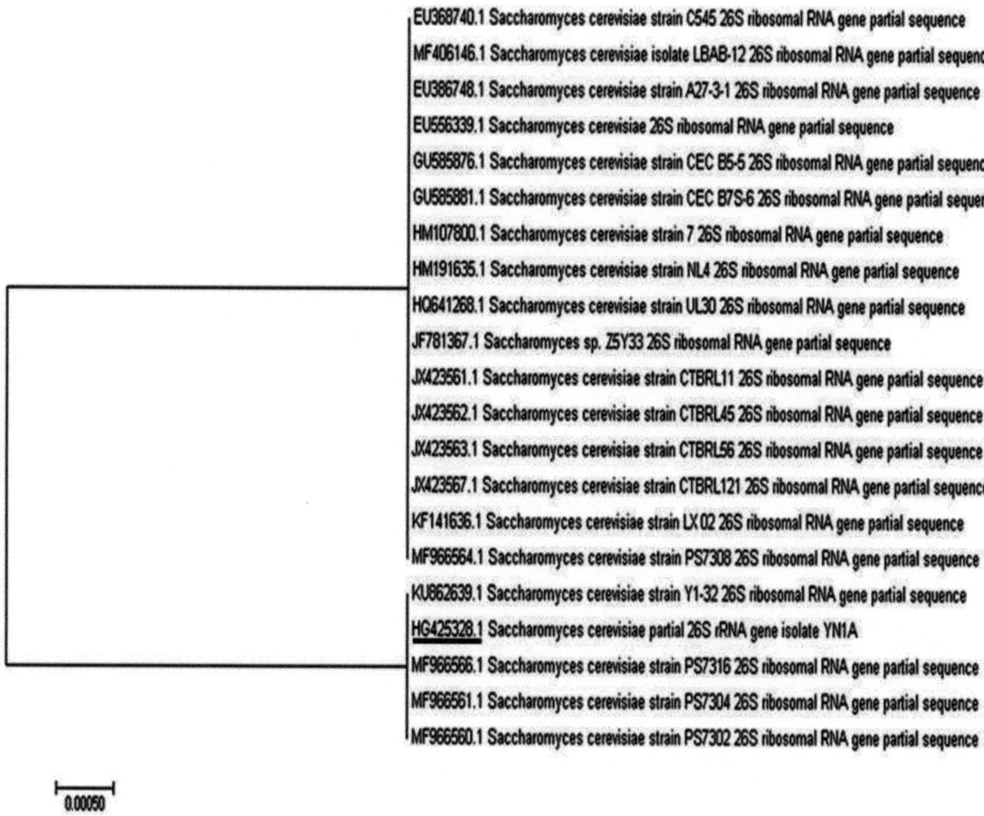

Figure 3. Phylogenetic analysis of *S. cerevisiae* (HG425328-underlined) from *Elaeis* sp. palm wine. The tree is drawn to scale, with branch lengths measured in the number of substitutions per site.

Saccharomyces sensu stricto and *Saccharomyces sensu lato* and the sensu stricto strains are mostly associated with the fermentation industry [43]. The *S. cerevisiae* in this study are *sensu stricto*. Comparative genomics analysis of *S. cerevisiae* and closely related species has contributed to our understanding of how new species emerge and has shed light on various mechanisms that contribute to reproductive isolation [44]. This knowledge can be applied to palm wine yeasts to ascertain how they differ from well characterized yeasts.

3.4. *Pichia kudriavzevii*

From recent molecular studies of yeasts present in palm wine, the yeast species *Pichia kudriavzevii* has emerged as a prevalent non-*Saccharomyces* yeast species in the drink. The genus has shown probiotic potentials [45] and multistress-tolerance [46]. It is worth looking closely at this genus because it has been shown that some *P. kudriavzevii* strains can produce higher quantities of ethanol from lignocellulosic biomass than conventional cells of *S. cerevisiae* at 45°C [47].

The tree constructed for *P. kudriavzevii* showed the least divergence when compared to *S. cerevisiae* or *Candida* palm wine yeast relatives. All the relatives and the *Elaeis* sp. palm wine strain (HG425333) originated from one node and formed separate taxonomic units

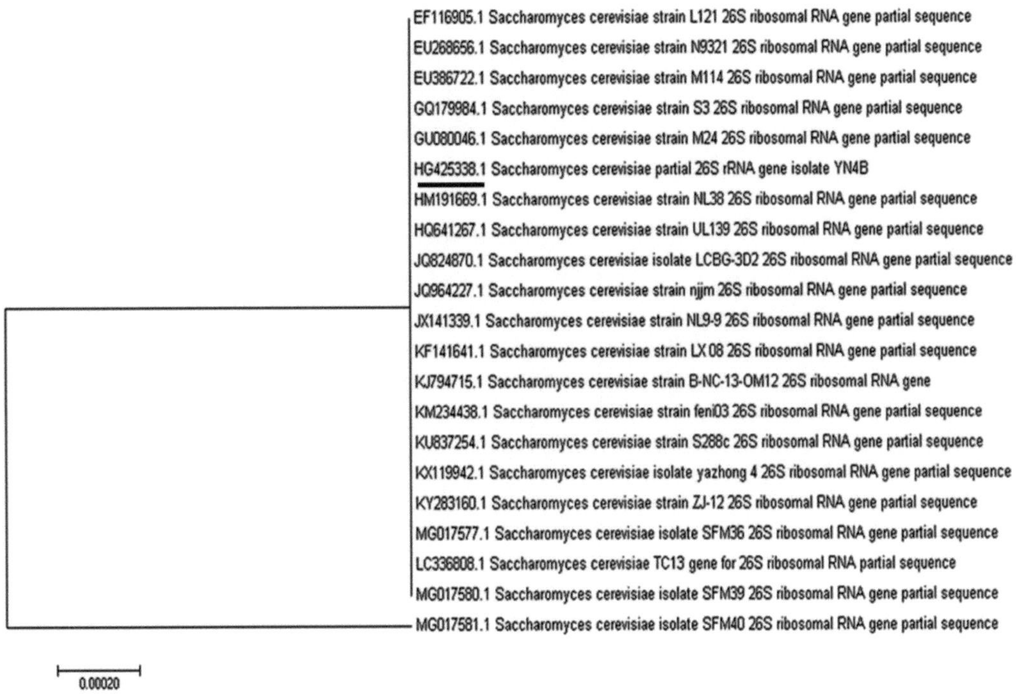

Figure 4. Phylogenetic analysis of *S. cerevisiae* (HG425338-underlined) from *Raphia* sp. palm wine. The tree is drawn to scale, with branch lengths measured in the number of substitutions per site.

(**Figure 5**). In contrast, the *P. kudriavzevii* (HG425335) from *Raphia* sp. palm wine formed a separate clade and did not lie on the same branch with the relatives (**Figure 6**). This indicates intraspecies diversity and confirms findings reported previously [11]. In that study, intraspecies diversity was suggested because *P. kudriavzevii* (HG425335) from *Raphia* sp. palm wine formed a separate clade with palm wine isolates from Mexico instead of isolates from the same geographical location.

The information contained in the sequence submission of close relatives of *P. kudriavzevii* strains also shows different sources of isolation. The strains close to the yeast from *Elaeis* sp. palm wine (HG425333, **Figure 5**) with accession numbers KY283159 and KM234455 show that isolation was from composite microbial powders for aquaculture [21] and naturally fermented cashew apple juice [48] whereas a close relative of *Raphia* sp. palm wine (HG425335, **Figure 6**) with accession number KU167717 was isolated from activated sludge from textile dyeing [49].

3.5. Geographical origin and sources of palm wine yeast relatives

After ascertaining the sources of very close relatives from the phylogenetic trees constructed, the shortlisted 600 sequences from the aforementioned yeast genera were further examined and the information found was used to group the isolates according to country of isolation, food, beverage, and non-edible source.

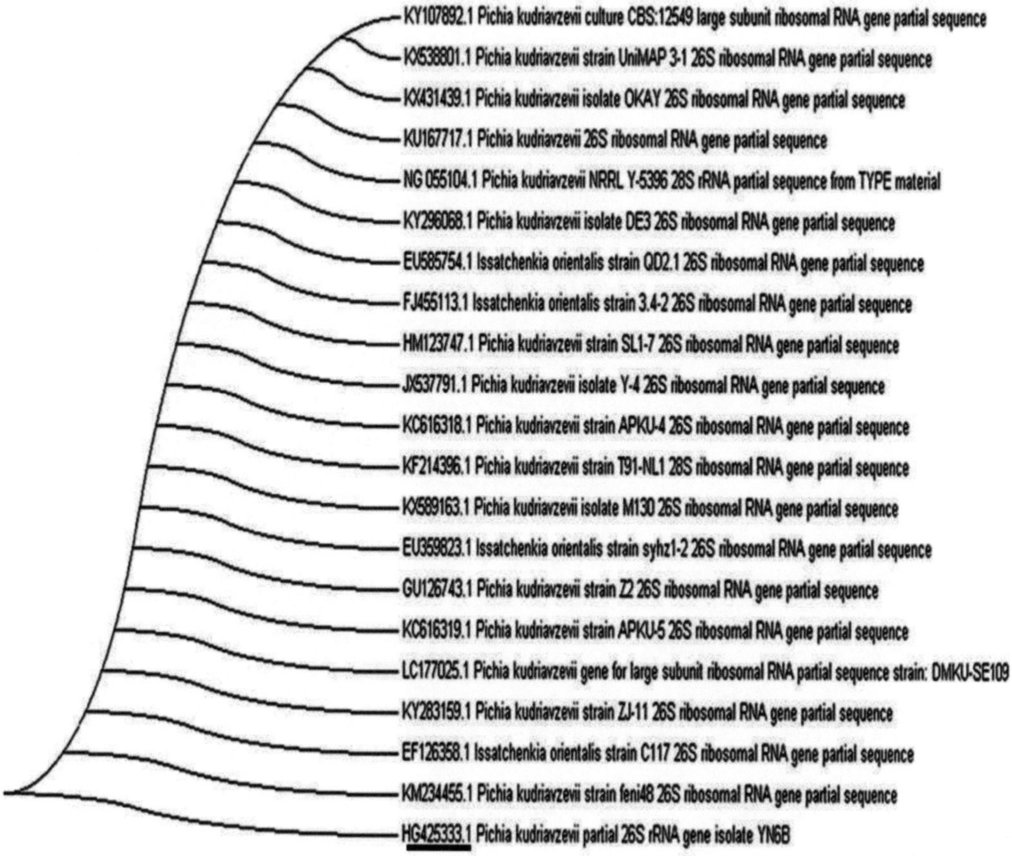

Figure 5. Phylogenetic analysis of *P. kudriavzevii* (HG425333-underlined) from *Elaeis* sp. palm wine. The tree is drawn to scale, with branch lengths measured in the number of substitutions per site.

3.5.1. Isolates submitted by country of origin and source

Overall, sequences examined for the aforementioned yeasts genera were submitted from 38 countries [18] and the top 6 countries is presented in this report. Sequence data for both *Elaeis* sp. (**Figure 7**) and *Raphia* sp. (**Figure 8**) palm trees show that highest number of submissions to the Genbank database was from China. The top three countries from which palm wine yeast relatives originated were the same for both palm tree species. This suggests that a large number of palm wine yeasts may have common ancestors with yeasts found in China. The origins or sources of palm wine yeasts relatives were spread across beverages, food, and non-food sources. The prevalence of *S. cerevisiae*, *P. kudriavzevii*, and *C. ethanolica* from these sources is shown for *Elaeis* sp. palm tree (**Figure 9**) and *Raphia* sp. palm tree (**Figure 10**). In both palm wine from *Elaeis* and *Raphia* palm trees, yeasts relatives of *S. cerevisiae* and *P. kudriavzevii* species were isolated mainly from beverage sources whereas relatives representing *C. ethanolica* species were isolated from non-food sources. The sources of isolation revealed that the closest relatives of palm wine yeasts were from various sources and not specific to any particular food or fermentation mix.

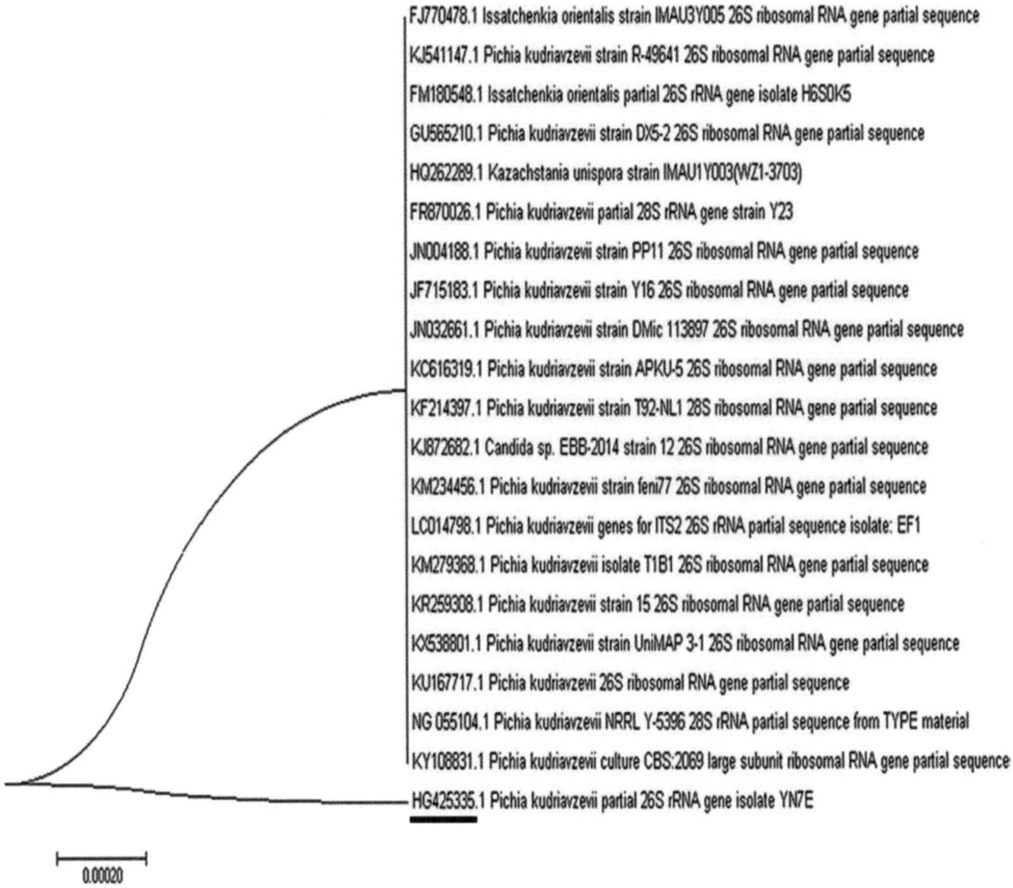

Figure 6. Phylogenetic analysis of *P. kudriavzevii* (HG425335-underlined) from *Raphia* sp. palm wine. The tree is drawn to scale, with branch lengths measured in the number of substitutions per site.

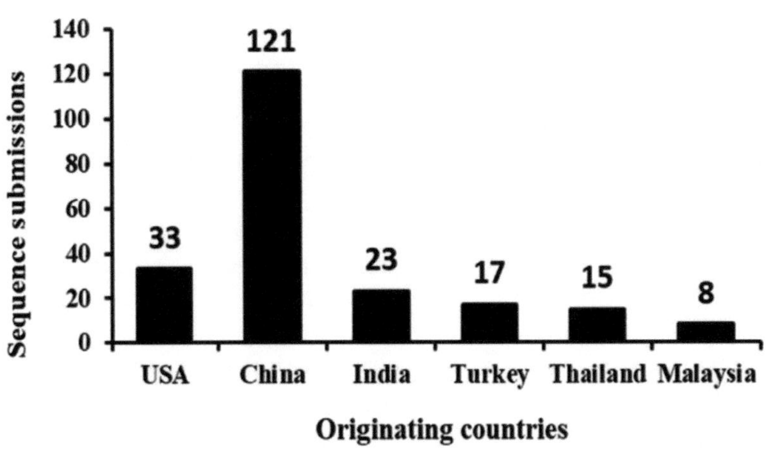

Figure 7. Top six countries from which sequences of palm wine yeast relatives of *Elaeis* sp. palm tree were submitted to the GenBank.

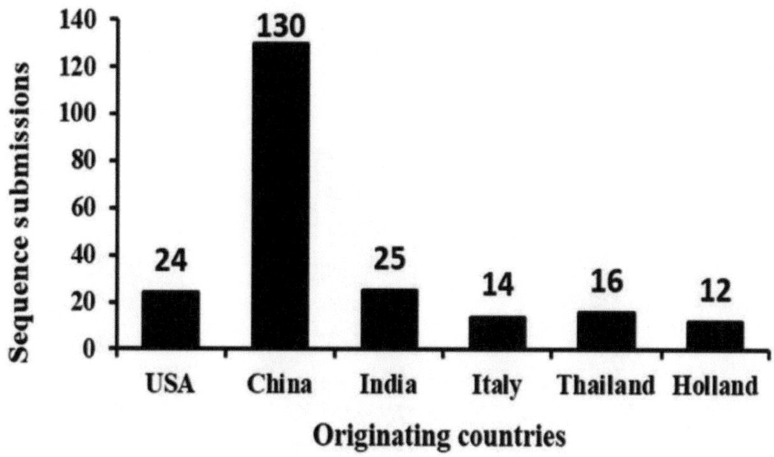

Figure 8. Top six countries from which sequences of palm wine yeast relatives of *Raphia* sp. palm tree were submitted to the GenBank.

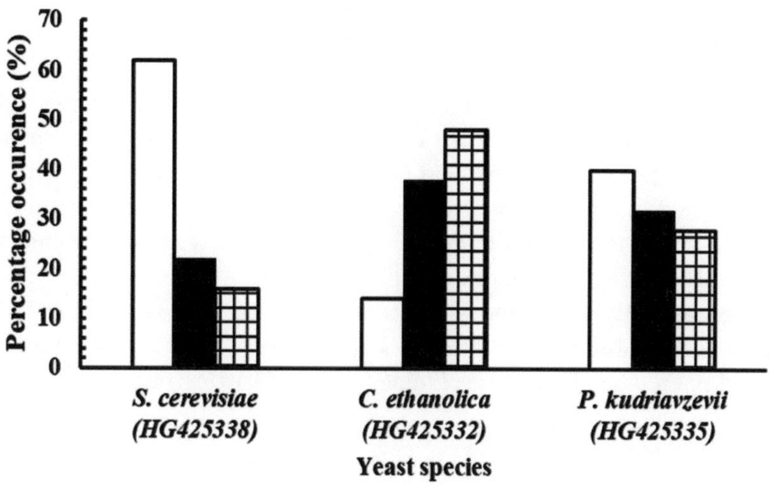

Figure 9. Distribution of palm wine yeast relatives with reference to yeasts from *Elaeis* sp. palm wine according to beverage (□), food (■), and non-food (⊞) sources.

A report [50] found that laboratory estimates of optimum growth temperature could be used to predict global distributions of free-living microbes. Also, it was pointed out that population genetic analyses show that the genetic diversity of *S. cerevisiae* is high in the tropics and subtropics of China [51, 52]. It was suggested that without further sampling in tropical and subtropical regions, it is not possible to differentiate whether the higher diversity of *S. cerevisiae* in Asia reflects a greater habitat area or an Asian origin for *S. cerevisiae*. It would be beneficial to carry out further studies in order to establish if palm wine yeasts were taken from Africa to Asia or vice versa. The diversity could also be high in temperate regions because a study examined *S. cerevisiae* and *S. paradoxus* in northeast America and uncovered a large diversity of yeasts [53]. Up to 24 yeast isolates could not be assigned to any known species and it was suggested that the yeasts identified may be of taxonomic, medical, or biotechnological importance.

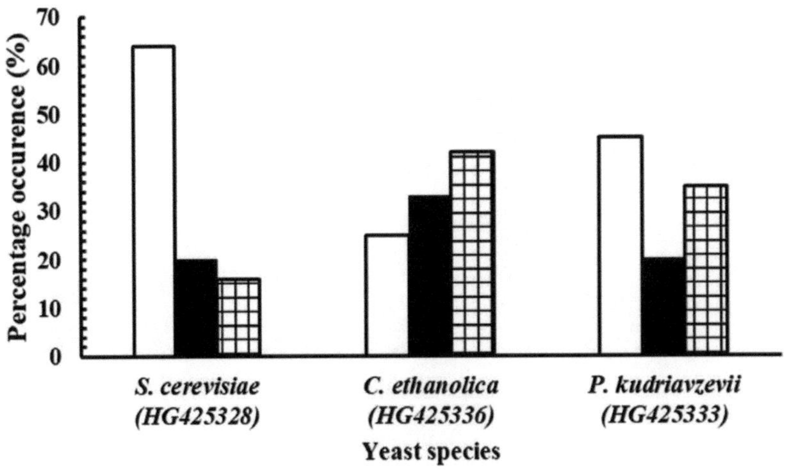

Figure 10. Distribution of palm wine yeast relatives with reference to yeasts from *Raphia* sp. palm wine according to beverage (□), food (▮), and non-food (⊞) sources.

3.6. G+C composition of palm wine yeast relatives

The G+C composition is a well known evolutionary property of eukaryotes, archaea, and bacteria. There are suggestions by Chen et al. [54], that concordance between proteomic architecture and the genetic code is related closely to genomic G+C content and phylogeny. It has been suggested that yeasts with higher G+C content have a higher recombination rate [55] and recombination is believed to be suppressed around centromeres [56]. The data in **Table 1** present the average nucleotide composition and G+C content of partial sequences of 26S rRNA genes analyzed. It shows concentration of arginine, guanine and thiamine, and cytosine concentration in *S. cerevisiae, P. kudriavzevii, or C. ethanolica* obtained from the aforementioned palm trees. Data were obtained after measuring nucleotide frequencies (%)

Yeast species	T/U	C	A	G	G+C
1. *S. cerevisiae*-R	26.3	16.6	26.5	30.7	47.3
2. *S. cerevisiae*-E	26.7	20.2	22.7	30.4	51.0
3. *P. kudriavzevii*-R	20.0	21.9	22.6	35.5	57.0
4. *P. kudriavzevii*-E	19.8	22.2	22.6	35.5	58.0
5. *C. ethanolica*-R	21.1	21.4	21.8	35.7	56.0
6. *C. ethanolica*-E	20.9	21.4	21.9	35.8	57.0

Nucleotide concentration was obtained after analysis with MEGA 7.0 software.
T/U, thiamine/uracil; C, cytosine; A, arginine; G, guanine.

Table 1. Average nucleotide composition and G+C content obtained from yeasts from *Raphia* sp. (R) or *Elaeis* sp. (E) palm wine and their relatives after measuring nucleotide frequencies (%) in 100 sequences relative to each yeast species shown.

in 100 sequences of strains relative to each palm wine yeast species listed. It was observed that the G+C content in *P. kudriavzevii* and *C. ethanolica* was higher than that of *S. cerevisiae*. This suggests that the *P. kudriavzevii* and *C. ethanolica* have a higher recombination rate than *S. cerevisiae* strains analyzed in this report. The G+C range observed is within the reported average genomic G+C-content range (13–75%) among species [57]. It was also found to be within range of G+C content (38.3–52.9%) of the *MAT* locus reported [58] in different *Saccharomycetaceae* species.

Further studies are required because G+C-content is associated with multiple biases of different nature during down stream operations and these biases may include sequencing technologies, biological, and methodological reasons [57]. Another factor that could affect the G+C content is that some yeasts like *Lachancea kluyveri* show an intriguing compositional heterogeneity in that a region of the chromosome has an average G+C content of 52.9% which is significantly higher than the 40.4% global G+C content of the rest of the genome [58].

4. Conclusions

Sequence data are useful for comparing palm wine yeasts from different trees. Data show the countries where the relatives of palm wine yeasts are dominant and may be useful for evolution and species migration studies. Palm wine yeast relatives may originate from beverage, food, and non-edible source. The G+C nucleotide data present insights on changes which may have occurred in conserved regions of some isolates over time. Comparing sequences with the highly conserved regions of the 26S rRNA genes gives an immediate picture of the lineage of palm wine yeasts and their relatives. It can also provide a foundation to select candidates for whole genome sequencing for comparision in future.

Acknowledgements

The free use of MEGA 7.0 is appreciated. Software can be accessed at https://www.megasoftware.net/home.

Author details

Ogueri Nwaiwu

Address all correspondence to: ogueri.nwaiwu@alpha-altis.co.uk

Alpha-Altis (Venture Member), Ingenuity Lab, The University of Nottingham, Nottingham, UK

References

[1] Reichgelt T, West CK, Greenwood DR. The relation between global palm distribution and climate. Scientific Report. 2018;**8**(4721):1-11

[2] Nwaiwu O, Ibekwe VI, Amadi ES, Udebuani AC, Nwanebu FC, Oguoma OI, Nnokwe JC. Evaluation of fermentation products of palm wine yeasts and role of *Sacoglottis gabonensis* supplement on products abundance. Beverages. 2016;**2**:1-13. DOI: 10.3390/beverages2020009

[3] Russell TA. The Raphia Palms of West Africa. Kew Bulletin. 1965;**19**(2):173-196

[4] Plant Use. *Raphia hookeri*—Plant resources of tropical Africa [Internet]. 2016. Available from: http://uses.plantnet-project.org/en/Raphia_hookeri_(PROTA) [Accessed: 2018-04-02]

[5] Food and Agricultural Organization. Origin of oil palm [Internet]. 2016. Available from: http://www.fao.org/DOCrEP/005/Y4355E/y4355e03.htm [Accessed: 2018-04-01]

[6] Legras JL, Merdinoglu D, Cornuet JM, Karst F. Bread, beer and wine: *Saccharomyces cerevisiae* diversity reflects human history. Molecular Ecology. 2007;**16**:2091-2102

[7] Tamang JP, Watanabe K, Holzapfel WH. Review: Diversity of microorganisms in global fermented foods and beverages. Frontiers in Microbiology. 2016;**7**:377. DOI: 10.3389/fmicb.2016.00377/

[8] Gallone B, Mertens S, Gordon JL, Maere S, Verstrepen KJ, Jan Steensels J. Origins, evolution, domestication and diversity of *Saccharomyces* beer yeasts. Current Opinion in Biotechnology. 2018;**49**:148-155

[9] Whitener MEB, Carlin S, Jacobson D, Weighill D, Divol B, Conterno L, du Toit M, Vrhovsek U. Early fermentation volatile metabolite profile of non-Saccharomyces yeasts in red and white grape must: A targeted approach. LWT Food Science and Technology. 2015;**64**:412-422

[10] Hittinger CT, Rokas A, Bai F-Y, Boekhout T, Gonçalves P, Jeffries TW, et al. Genomics and the making of yeast biodiversity. Current Opinion in Genetics and Development. 2015;**35**:100-109

[11] Nwaiwu O, Itumoh M. Molecular phylogeny of yeasts from palm wine and enological potentials of the drink. Annual Research and Review in Biology. 2017;**20**:1-12. DOI: 10.9734/ARRB/2017/37748

[12] Nwaiwu O. Use of fragments from D1/D2 Domain of 26S rRNA gene to select *Saccharomyces cerevisiae* from palm wine. Journal of Applied Life Sciences International. 2016;**5**:1-5. DOI: 10.9734/JALSI/2016/26373

[13] Kannan L, Wheeler WC. Maximum parsimony on phylogenetic networks, algorithms. Molecular Biology. 2012;**7**:1-10. DOI: 10.1186/1748-7188-7-9

[14] Kumar S, Stecher G, Tamura K. MEGA7: Molecular evolutionary genetics analysis version 7.0 for bigger datasets. Molecular Biology and Evolution. 2016;**33**:1870-1874

[15] Edgar RC. MUSCLE: Multiple sequence alignment with high accuracy and high throughput. Nucleic Acids Research. 2004;**32**:1792-1797

[16] Tamura K, Nei M. Estimation of the number of nucleotide substitutions in the control region of mitochondrial DNA in humans and chimpanzees. Molecular Biology and Evolution. 1993;**10**:512-526

[17] Tamura K. Estimation of the number of nucleotide substitutions when there are strong transition-transversion and G+C-content biases. Molecular Biology and Evolution. 1992;**9**:678-687

[18] Nwaiwu O. Sequence and alignment data on yeasts from palm wine and their relatives. figshare [Internet]. 2018. Available from: https://doi.org/10.6084/m9.figshare.6496676.v1 [Accessed: 2018-06-13]

[19] Steensels J, Verstrepen KJ. Taming Wild Yeast: Potential of conventional and non-conventional yeasts in industrial fermentations. Annual Review of Microbiology. 2014;**68**:61-80

[20] Zhou N, Katz M, Knecht W, Compagno C, Piškur J. Genome dynamics and evolution in yeasts: A long-term yeast-bacteria competition experiment. PLoS ONE. 2018;**13**(4):e0194911. DOI: 10.1371/journal.pone.0194911

[21] Altschul SF, Gish W, Miller W, Myers EW, Lipman DJ. Basic local alignment search tool. Journal of Molecular Biology. 1990;**215**:403-410

[22] Benson DA, Karsch-Mizrachi I, Clark K, Lipman DJ, Ostell J, Eric W, Sayers EW. Genbank. Nucleic Acids Research. 2017;**45**(Database issue):D37-D42. DOI: 10.1093/nar/gkw1070

[23] National Center for Biotechnology Information Phylogenetic Resources [Internet]. https://www.ncbi.nlm.nih.gov/Class/NAWBIS/Modules/Phylogenetics/phylo15.html [Accessed: 2018-06-20]

[24] Mukherjee M, Radecka D, Aerts G, Verstrepen KJ, Lievens B, Thevelein JM. Phenotypic landscape of non-conventional yeast species for different stress tolerance traits desirable in bioethanol fermentation. Biotechnology for Biofuels. 2017;**10**:216

[25] Steensels J, Daenen L, Malcorps P, Derdelinck G, Verachtert H, Verstrepen KJ. Brettanomyces yeasts—From spoilage organisms to valuable contributors to industrial fermentations. International Journal of Food Microbiology. 2015;**206**:24-38

[26] Zhao J. Molecular identifiation of strains isolated from composite microbial powders for aquaculture [Internet]. 2016. Available from: https://www.ncbi.nlm.nih.gov/nuccore/ky283163 [Accessed: 2018-03-01]

[27] Nielsen DS, Teniola OD, Ban-Koffi L, Owusu M, Andersson TS, Holzapfel WH. The microbiology of Ghanaian cocoa fermentations analysed using culture-dependent and culture-independent methods. International Journal of Food Microbiology. 2007;**114**:168-186

[28] Wang H. Yeasts associated with aerobic deterioration in total mixed ration silage [Internet]. 2016. Available from: https://www.ncbi.nlm.nih.gov/nuccore/km005182 [Accessed: 2018-03-03]

[29] Kurtzman CP, Robnett CJ. Identification and phylogeny of ascomycetous yeasts from analysis of nuclear large subunit (26S) ribosomal DNA partial sequences. Antonie Van Leeuwenhoek. 1998;**73**:331-371

[30] Kanpiengjai A, Khanongnuch C. Distribution of tannin tolerant yeasts associated with naturally fermented *Miang* leaves, *Camellia sinensis var. assamica* in northern Thailand [Internet]. 2016. Available from: https://www.ncbi.nlm.nih.gov/nuccore/kx055483 [Accessed: 2018-04-03]

[31] Vu D, Groenewald M, Szoke S, Cardinali G, Eberhardt U, Stielow B, et al. DNA barcoding analysis of more than 9000 yeast isolates contributes to quantitative thresholds for yeast species and genera delimitation. Studies in Mycology. 2016;**85**:91-105

[32] Brandt ME, Lockhart SR. Recent taxonomic developments with *Candida* and other opportunistic yeasts. Current Fungal Infection Reports. 2012;**6**:170-177

[33] Mühlhause S, Kollmar M. Molecular phylogeny of sequenced *Saccharomycetes* reveals polyphyly of the alternative yeast codon usage. Genome Biology and Evolution. 2014;**6**:3222-3237

[34] Hawksworth DL. A new dawn for the naming of fungi: Impacts of decisions made in Melbourne in July 2011 on the future publication and regulation of fungal names. Mycokeys. 2011;**1**:7-20

[35] Robert V, Vu D, Amor ABH, van de Wiele N, Brouwer C, Jabas B, et al. MycoBank gearing up for new horizons. IMA Fungus. 2013;**4**:371-379

[36] Duina AA, Miller ME, Keeney JB. Budding yeast for budding geneticists: A primer on the *Saccharomyces cerevisiae* model systemnetics. Genetics. 2014;**197**:33-48

[37] Brice C, Cubillos FA, Dequin S, Camarasa C, Martínez C. Adaptability of the *Saccharomyces cerevisiae* yeasts to wine fermentation conditions relies on their strong ability to consume nitrogen. PLoS One. 2018;**13**(2):e0192383. DOI: 10.1371/journal.pone.0192383

[38] Liu Y, Jiao J. Regional differences of grape-surface microbes significantly influence the melatonin level of wine during fermentation [Internet]. 2016. Available from: https://www.ncbi.nlm.nih.gov/nuccore/KU862639 [Accessed: 2018-05-03]

[39] Yu Y. *Saccharomyces cerevisiae* strain PS7316 26S ribosomal RNA gene, partial sequence [Internet]. 2017. Available from: https://www.ncbi.nlm.nih.gov/nuccore/mf966566 [Accessed: 2018-05-03]

[40] Zhang J. Molecular identification of wine yeasts [Internet]. 2016. Available from: https://www.ncbi.nlm.nih.gov/nuccore/gu080046 [Accessed: 2018-05-04]

[41] Zhu LX, Zhang LL, Gong MF. Analysis of 26S rDNA sequences of yeasts isolated from Musalais grape wine [Internet]. 2010. Available from: https://www.ncbi.nlm.nih.gov/nuccore/hm191669 [Accessed: 2018-05-06]

[42] Barriga EJC, Libkind D, Briones AI, Iranzo JU, Portero P, Roberts I, James S, Morais PB, Rosa CA. Yeasts biodiversity and its significance: Case studies in natural and human-related environments, ex situ preservation, applications and challenges [Internet]. 2011. Available

from: http://www.intechopen.com/books/changing-diversity-in-changing-environment/yeastsbiodiversity-and-its-significance-case-studies-in-natural-and-human-related-environments-ex-s [Accessed: 2018-05-08]

[43] Imanishi Y, Ueda-Nishimura K, Mikata K. Two newspecies of *Kazachstania* that form ascospores connected bya belt-like intersporal body: *Kazachstania zonata* and *Kazachstania gamospora*. FEMS Yeast Research. 2007;**7**:330-338

[44] Marsit S, Leducq J-B, Durand E, Marchant A, Filteau M, Landry CR. Evolutionary biology through the lens of budding yeast comparative genomics. Nature Reviews Genetics. 2017;**18**:581-598

[45] Greppi A, Saubade F, Botta C, Humblot C, Guyot JP, Cocolin L. Potential probiotic *Pichia kudriavzevii* strains and their ability to enhance folate content of traditional cereal-based African fermented food. Food Microbiology. 2017;**62**:169-177

[46] Bae J, Han J, Jeong H, Ko H, Park H, Sohn J, Sung B. Draft genome sequence of a multistress-tolerant yeast, *Pichia kudriavzevii* NG7. Genome Announcement. 2018;**6**: e01515-e01517

[47] Oberoi HS, Babbar N, Sandhu SK, Dhaliwal SS, Kaur U, Chadha BS, Bhargav VK. Ethanol production from alkali-treated rice straw via simultaneous saccharification and fermentation using newly isolated thermotolerant *Pichia kudriavzevii* HOP-1. Journal of Industrial Microbiology and Biotechnology. 2012;**39**:557-566

[48] Prabhu-Khorjuvenka SN, Doijad SP, Barbuddhe SB. Diversity of yeasts isolated from naturally fermented cashew apple juice [Internet]. 2014. Available from: https://www.ncbi.nlm.nih.gov/nuccore/km234455 [Accessed: 2018-05-07]

[49] Rosu C, Stefan A. Biodegradation of azo dyes by ascomycete yeasts [Internet]. 2017. Available from: https://www.ncbi.nlm.nih.gov/nuccore/ku167717 [Accessed: 2018-05-07]

[50] Robinson HA, Pinharanda A, Bensasson D. Summer temperature can predict the distribution of wild yeast populations. Ecology and Evolution. 2016;**6**:1236-1250

[51] Wang QM, Liu WQ, Liti G, Wang SA, Bai FY. Surprisingly diverged populations of *Saccharomyces cerevisiae* in natural environments remote from human activity. Molecular Ecology. 2012;**21**:5404-5417

[52] Almeida P, Barbosa R, Zalar P, Imanishi Y, Shimizu K, Turchetti B, et al. A population genomics insight into the Mediterranean origins of wine yeast domestication. Molecular Ecology. 2015;**24**:5412-5427

[53] Charron G, Leducq J-P, Bertin C, Dubé AK, Landry LR. Exploring the northern limit of the distribution of *Saccharomyces cerevisiae* and *Saccharomyces paradoxus* in North America. FEMS Yeast Research. 2014;**14**:281-288

[54] Chen W, Yanchun Shao Y, Fusheng CF. Evolution of complete proteomes: Guanine-cytosine pressure, phylogeny and environmental influences blend the proteomic architecture. BMC Evolutionary Biology. 2013;**13**:21. DOI: https://doi.org/10.1186/1471-2148-13-219

[55] Bradnam KR, Seoighe C, Sharp PM, Wolfe KH. G+C content variation along and among *Saccharomyces cerevisiae* chromosomes. Molecular Biology and Evolution. 1999;**16**:666-675

[56] Lynch DB, Logue ME, Butler G, Wolfe KH. Chromosomal G+C content evolution in yeasts: Systematic interspecies differences, and GC-poor troughs at centromeres. Genome Biology and Evolution. 2010;**2**:572-583

[57] Romiguier J, Roux C. Analytical biases associated with GC-content in molecular evolution. Frontiers in Genetics. 2017;**8**:16. DOI: 10.3389/fgene.2017.00016

[58] Payen C, Fischer G, Marck C, Proux C, Sherman DJ, Coppe'e J-Y, Johnston M, Dujon B, Neuveglise C. Unusual composition of a yeast chromosome arm is associated with its delayed replication. Genome Research. 2009;**19**:1710-1721

Chapter 3

Importance of Molecular and Phylogenetic Analyses for Identification of Basidiomycetes

Samina Sarwar, Qudsia Firdous and
Abdul Nasir Khalid

Additional information is available at the end of the chapter

http://dx.doi.org/10.5772/intechopen.80671

Abstract

Fungi are considered as diverse group of eukaryotic organisms and have very important role in ecosystem. Although their expected number is more than 2.2–3.8 million, only 120,000 taxa have been identified so far. Basidiomycetes are very large group of fungi including mushrooms, toad stools, puff balls, earth stars, polypores, and rust and smut fungi. Previously, these fungi were identified only by morphological characters that have been considered as variable due to environmental factors. Literature shows that many fungi are misidentified due to phenotypic changes. Molecular methods including phylogenetics prove to be successful aids along with traditional methods for correct identification of these fungi and these have revolutionized fungal reclassification. Many fungal taxa have been shifted to other groups of fungi after their phylogenetic analysis. So, many DNA markers can be used to solve such problems.

Keywords: Agaricales, morphology, mushrooms, primers, systematic

1. Introduction

1.1. Basidiomycetes

In biologist opinion, relationship of phylogenetics can be the dominant support of research in different areas of biology. The most expressing visions into biology are through species comparisons and phylogenetic analysis of gene sequence background. Its importance can be seen in diverse subfields including physiology, ecology, and molecular biology [1, 2].

IntechOpen

© 2019 The Author(s). Licensee IntechOpen. This chapter is distributed under the terms of the Creative Commons Attribution License (http://creativecommons.org/licenses/by/3.0), which permits unrestricted use, distribution, and reproduction in any medium, provided the original work is properly cited.

The largest groups of fungi (Basidiomycetes) including many mushrooms, some are edible, have become more significant in recent times for their nutritional and medicinal properties. It is the second largest group of fungi that produce sexual basidiospores in modified cell called the basidium. This class has the resemblance with animal, plants, red and green algae, several groups of slime molds, water molds (oomycetes), brown algae, Ascomycetes (including lichens), and Phycomycetes (Glomeromycetes, Zygomycetes, and Chytridiomycetes) due to the presence of some important similar characters [3].

There are more than 30,000 species in Basidiomycota, and this number is increasing day by day [4]. More specifically, this division of characterization can be portrayed under the number of request of gilled and nongilled fungi [5]. Mueller and his companions [6] exhibited the aggregate expected number of gilled fungi around 80,000; out of which just 13,000 are known yet and these are extremely basic segment of forests, either on rotting wood and other dead plant material as saprotrophs or symbionts with the living cells of plant roots, forming mycorrhizal associations with trees, others are parasites on living plants [7].

1.2. Classification of Basidiomycetes

Basidiomycetes are categorized into rusts, smuts, Heterobasidiomycetes, Homobasidiomycetes, Gasteromycetes, Hymenomycetes, Dacrymycetales, Agaricales, and Aphyllophorales [8].

2. Methods

2.1. Cataloging techniques for Basidiomycete identification

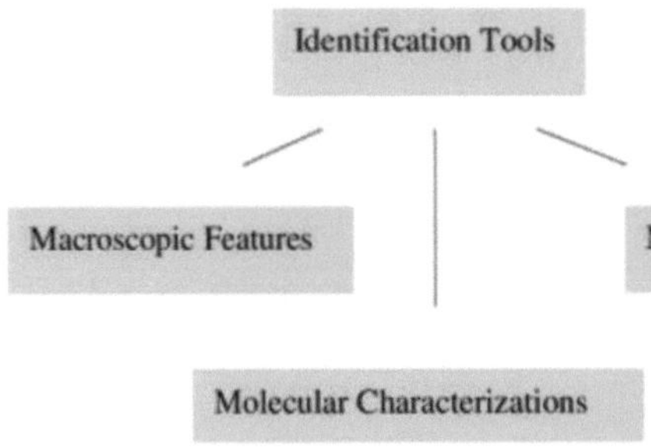

Basically, scientists use three different markers for Basidiomycete identification including macroscopic, microscopic, and molecular analyses.

2.1.1. Macroscopic features for Basidiomycete identification

To be arranged appropriately, valid recognizable proof is required. There are numerous conventional techniques for distinguishing proof of these fungi, yet not every one of them are solid and reliable [9, 10]. Prior, the gilled fungi were recognized and named based on certain macroscopic features, that is, longevity, texture, color of internal tissues, form, spore and basidia bearing surface, dimensions, host and nature of deterioration accompanying with a sporocarp on wood. Generally, Basidiomycetes (mostly mushrooms) are identified morphologically by their spore print color, ring and volva on stipe (presence/absence), substrate type, surface texture, and gill/hymenium attachment to the stipe. As we can observe that all these characters are variable to some extent with environmental conditions and cannot be used as prime features for identification purpose [11] (**Figure 1**).

2.1.2. Microscopic features for Basidiomycete identification

Traditionally, microscopic features are also used for the identification of these fungi [11]. Microscopic characters taken into consideration by many scientists include (a) hyphal composition of basidioma tissues which are of three types *viz.*, generative, skeletal, and binding hyphae. These hyphae form three different types of basidioma monomitic, dimitic, or trimitic; (b) nature of hymenium, basidia, cystidia, basidiospores, their shapes, dimensions, and color reaction in different reagents, and (c) clamp connections (presence/absence) [12] (**Figure 2**).

2.1.3. Misleading identification factors

The taxonomy of Basidiomycetes has been controversial because of the limited number of distinguish morphological characters, and there is uncertainty for sorting out of different sections and species. Environmental factors and substrate have great influence on phenotypic variation may cause troublesome in morphological identification of edible mushroom. One of the major issues for mushroom reproducers is the absence of an orderly consensus contrivance to segregate diverse species, which are occasionally morphologically indistinguishable [13].

Hence, they have to build up a proper strategy for distinguishing taxa [14]. The implements of molecular approaches are essential to confirm species delimitation. Traditional morphological strategies are less credible than cutting edge techniques that give more dependable approaches to distinguishing proof.

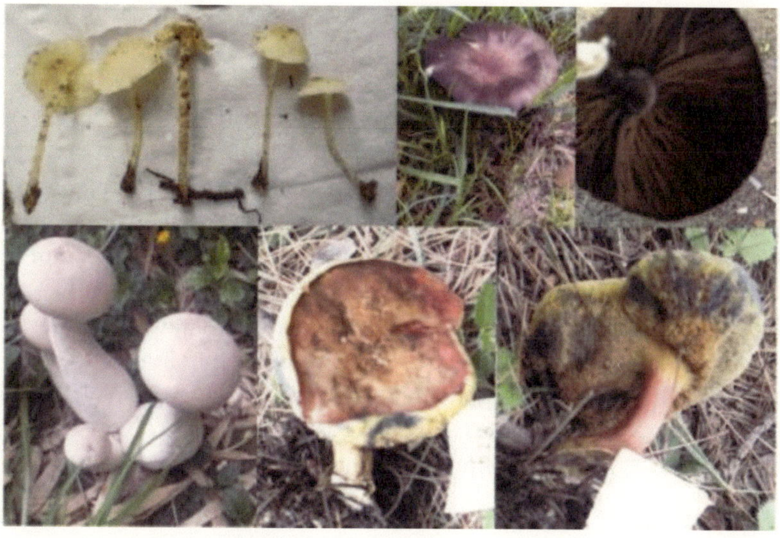

Figure 1. Some Basidiomycetes showing different morphological characters. The photos in the figure are the original collection by the authors of this chapter from Pakistan.

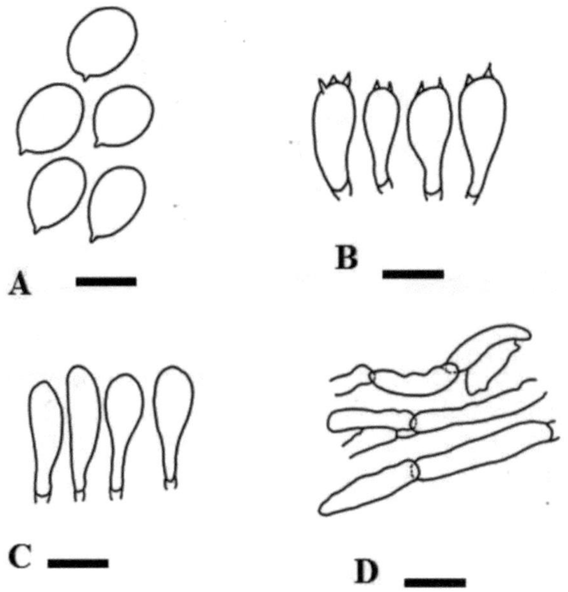

Figure 2. Different microscopic features of Basidiomycetes. (A) Basidiospores, (B) Basidia, (C) Cystidia, and (D) Pileipellis. These are the line drawings (anatomical structures) of *Agaricus* spp. prepared by the authors.

3. Advanced molecular methods for Basidiomycete identification

3.1. Molecular techniques

The recent improvement in DNA technology has been regarded as a prerequisite procedure provided a powerful addition to traditional taxonomic methods. Due to the limitations of conventional methods, molecular techniques are used to investigate the problems related to identification and classification of species. For fungal diagnosis, a high variety of molecular methods are progressively becoming important tools in all aspects for identification. There are several advanced level techniques that can be used for the identification of these fungi [15]. However, the use of DNA marker is base for all methods which provide connection between unknown fungi and fully described, morphologically characterized herbarium specimen. Fungal identification is somewhat dependent upon reference species that have been identified by mycological taxonomist for specific class of fungi that was taken into consideration with appropriate skills. Additional sources of information can be obtained from public DNA sequence databases for tentative identifications but should not totally relied upon these database sequences, as authenticating the distinctiveness of source material is rarely possible. Important molecular techniques include Southern blotting, PCR restriction fragment length polymorphism (PCR-RFLP), RAPD, PCR, DNA sequencing, microarrays, etc. DNA extraction and purification is the first step for any of these methods, for which many protocols and prepared kits are existing [16].

In fungal categorization, DNA strategies are fast and authentic to build up the individualities of wild collections. After the approach of cycle sequencing technique [16], direct sequencing of PCR products turned into a normal issue at least in organelle DNA loci or repetitive nuclear

DNA such as ribosomal DNAs [17]. This innovation is thought to be a standout among the most great techniques for phylogenetic investigations [18, 19]. Internal transcribed spacer (ITS) region of rDNA is usually utilized region for molecular recognizable proof of Basidiomycetes growing in differing natural surroundings. The corelationship among phenotypes and genotypes has been archived as phylogeny [20].

3.2. Fungal barcoding

A barcode is a categorization of a definite country of the genome which encompasses approximately genetic discrepancy among species, so countenancing one species to be renowned from an additional. The foremost DNA section which encounters this criterion for fungi is the "nuclear ribosomal internal transcribed spacer" or (ITS) expanse. Fungal DNA covers manifold copies of the ITS region which safeguards a virtuous resource of appropriate substantial for abstraction and examination. The barcode regions jumble-sale for fungal taxonomy characteristically ranges from 400 to 1000 base pairs in distance. Comprehensive studies which engender phylogenetic trees customarily expenditure arrangement evidence from supplementary than one barcode region. A barcode for an unidentified/unfamiliar species can be paralleled with barcodes apprehended in intercontinental records including GenBank and UNITE. Conversely, inaccuracies such as imprecisions in credentials of the original material or certification errors at a later date cast doubt on the validity of some records. A study by [21] nominated that more than 27% of all fungal ITS sequences were insufficiently identified in the International Nucleotide Sequence Database and in many cases had "compromised taxonomic annotations" [22].

3.2.1. Choice of primer

Choice of primer is a very crucial step. Nevertheless, one should start amplifying the ITS region of Basidiomycetes because of two reasons: first of all, universal primer for fungi (ITS1F) can work on it favorably, and secondly, this region has occupied maximum data of all type of fungi, incomparable to other barcoding regions which are now being the interest of scientist (Mycologist). Especially in the case of nom. prov. (seems new) species where data based on one genetic region seems insufficient and unreliable. Moreover, the most suitable primer will be chosen according to the category of a Basidiomycete to which it belongs to. Mostly, universal primer for fungi, that is, ITS1F is used as a forward primer that reads from 5′ to 3′ direction of one template strand, while ITS4 is being used as reverse primer that reads the second template DNA strand from 3′ to 5′ direction. There are many other fungal specified primers that have been used for different groups of fungi [9] (**Figures 3** and **4**).

3.2.2. Fungal barcoding primers

Following are some important primers that are under the use for molecular and phylogenetic study of Basidiomycetes.

- ITS Primers: ITS1, ITS2, ITS3, ITS1F, ITS4, ITS8-F, ITS6-R, ITS4BR, ITS4BR2, ITS3R2, ITS242, ITS5, ITS3R3, 5.8S, 5.8SR, UN-UP18S42, UN-LO28S22, BE1, and BE2.
- LSU Primers: LR0R, LR5, and LR16.
- SSU Primers: SR1R, NS1, NSR, PNS1, and NS41.

- RPB1Primers: RPB1-Af, RPB1-Ac, and RPB1-Cr.
- RPB2 Primers: fRBb2-5F, RPB2-7R, and Brpb2-7.1R.
- MCM7 Primers: Mcm7-709for, Mcm7-1348rev, and Mcm7-1447rev.

3.2.3. Phylogenetics

Phylogenetics is the learning of evolutionary associations among biological bodies often genes, individual or species and assists to classify the organism, finding pathogenies, forensic sciences or in bioinformatics. Sometimes, it provides base line to investigate the fundamental relationships among different taxa belonging to whether same or different class, while most of the time, it also helps in approaching application of a particular morphon [23].

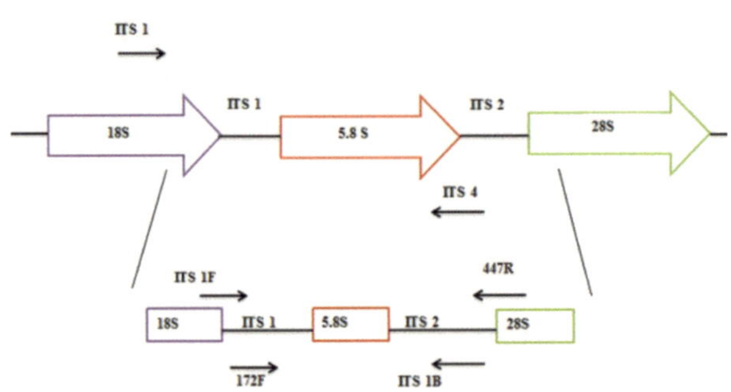

Figure 3. Internal specified region of a part of genome. © Mishra RK, Verma DK, Pandey BK, Pathak N and Zeeshan M (2014) Direct Colony Nested-PCR for the Detection of Fusarium oxysporum f. sp. Psidii Causing Wilt Disease in Psidium guajava L. J Horticulture 1:105. doi:10.4172/2376-0354.1000105.

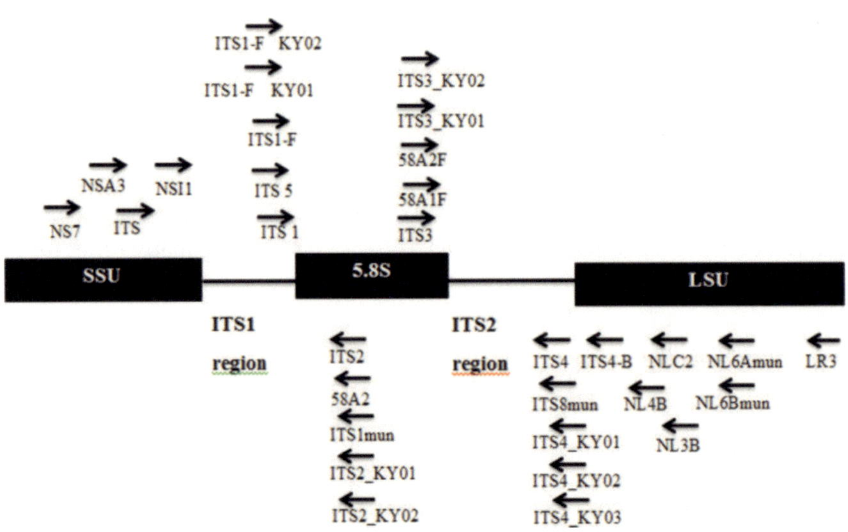

Figure 4. Three regions and their directions to amplify. © Toju H, Tanabe AS, Yamamoto S, Sato H (2012) High-Coverage ITS Primers for the DNA-Based Identification of Ascomycetes and Basidiomycetes in Environmental Samples. PLoS ONE 7(7): e40863. https://doi.org/10.1371/journal.pone.0040863 credited.

4. Results and discussion

4.1. Example for basidiocarp identification (problem solving)

Entoloma rhodopolium is a poisonous species causes gastrointestinal diseases, and muscarine, muscardine, and choline have also been insulated as noxious mediators. It is commonly known as wood pink gill often confused with morphologically similar species *E. sarcopum* (edible). To save someone's life, correct and authentic identification is very much necessary here. Hence, finally phylogenetic investigation of *E. rhodopolium* was accompanied by using RPB2 and ITS sequences, and the result was matched with that of previously described species from Europe making three clades. Based on the taxonomy, a simple proof for the identification technique, PCR-RFLP was followed to distinguish between edible *E. sarcopum* and poisonous species which was actual parallel in morphology. The learning can provide assistance to elucidate the classification of complex *E. rhodopolium*-related species, and to take avoiding action from food poisoning [17] (**Figure 5**).

Similarly, Nawaz et al. [24] carried out a research to identify *Melanoleuca* species from Pakistan. Only morphological parameters cannot help to identify of *Melanoleuca* species [25, 26], and so, their identification mainly depends on phylogenetic analyses [27]. *Melanoleuca dirensis* is distinct from the other taxa in the subgenus based on the morphoanatomical and phylogenetic characters. Although, the size of the stipe and lageniform cystidia are shared characters between *M. cinereifolia* and *M. dirensis*, *M. dirensis* differs from *M. cinereifolia* in having white lamellae and fusoid-ventricose cheilocystidia, while *M. cinereifolia* bears gray lamellae [25, 27]. *Melanoleuca dirensis*, a new species from Pakistan [24] belonging to above mentioned genus was identified by phylogenetic tree analyses.

4.2. Example for ectomycorrhizal morphotype identification

Ectomycorrhizal association of Basidiomycetes is an important part of any ecosystem for trees growth which leads toward increase in forestry. Previously, ectomycorrhizal morphotypes

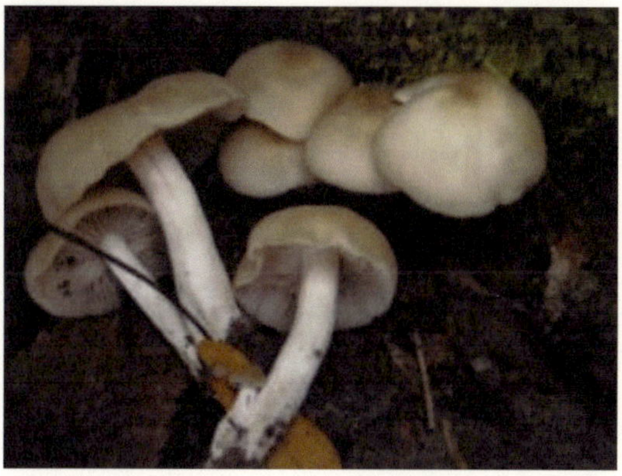

Figure 5. *Entoloma rhodopolium* (copyright) of Michael Kuo (Kuo, M. (2014, January). *Entoloma rhodopolium*. Retrieved from the MushroomExpert.Com).

were identified by morphotyping methods [28]. No doubt, characters for morphotyping are important for the identification and taxonomic purpose, but some time these characters mislead in identification [29] due to similar characters in different morphotypes and different characters of same species morphotypes when their host tree is different. Molecular and phylogenetic analyses resolve this problem. Now mycologists can easily identify mycobiont as well as phycobiont by using such advanced methods. Corresponding author of this chapter has identified many mycobionts from Himalayan range of Pakistan by using molecular methods [30–34]. Following phylogenetic trees are two examples among these. **Figure 6** explains ectomycorrhizal morphotypes of *Suillus flavidus*. These morphotypes were isolated from rhizosphere of conifers from Pakistan and were tried to identify by morphotyping methods, but ultimate identification was possible only by molecular and phylogenetic analyses [32]. Similarly, **Figure 7** explains mycobiont of another mushroom *Suillus himalayensis*,

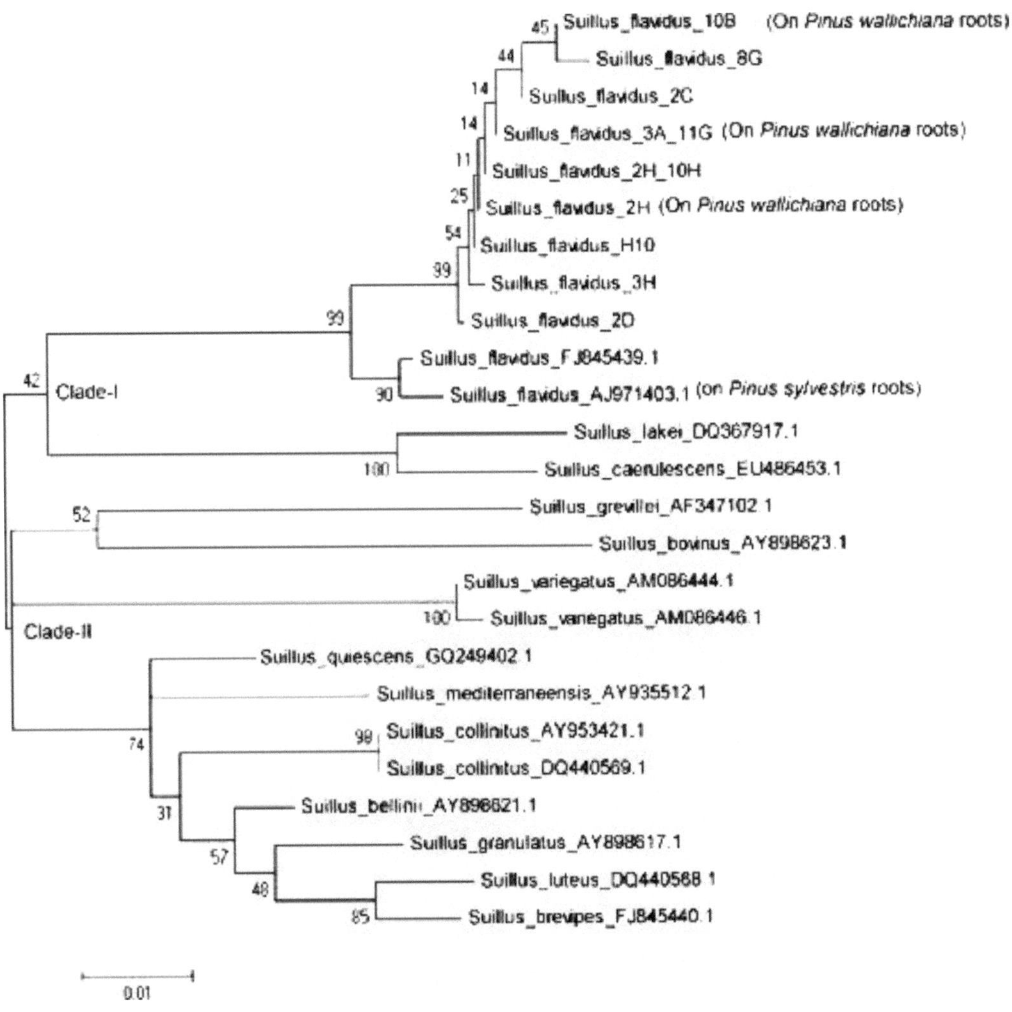

Figure 6. Phylogenetic analyses of ectomycorrhizal morphotypes of *Suillus flavidus* [32].

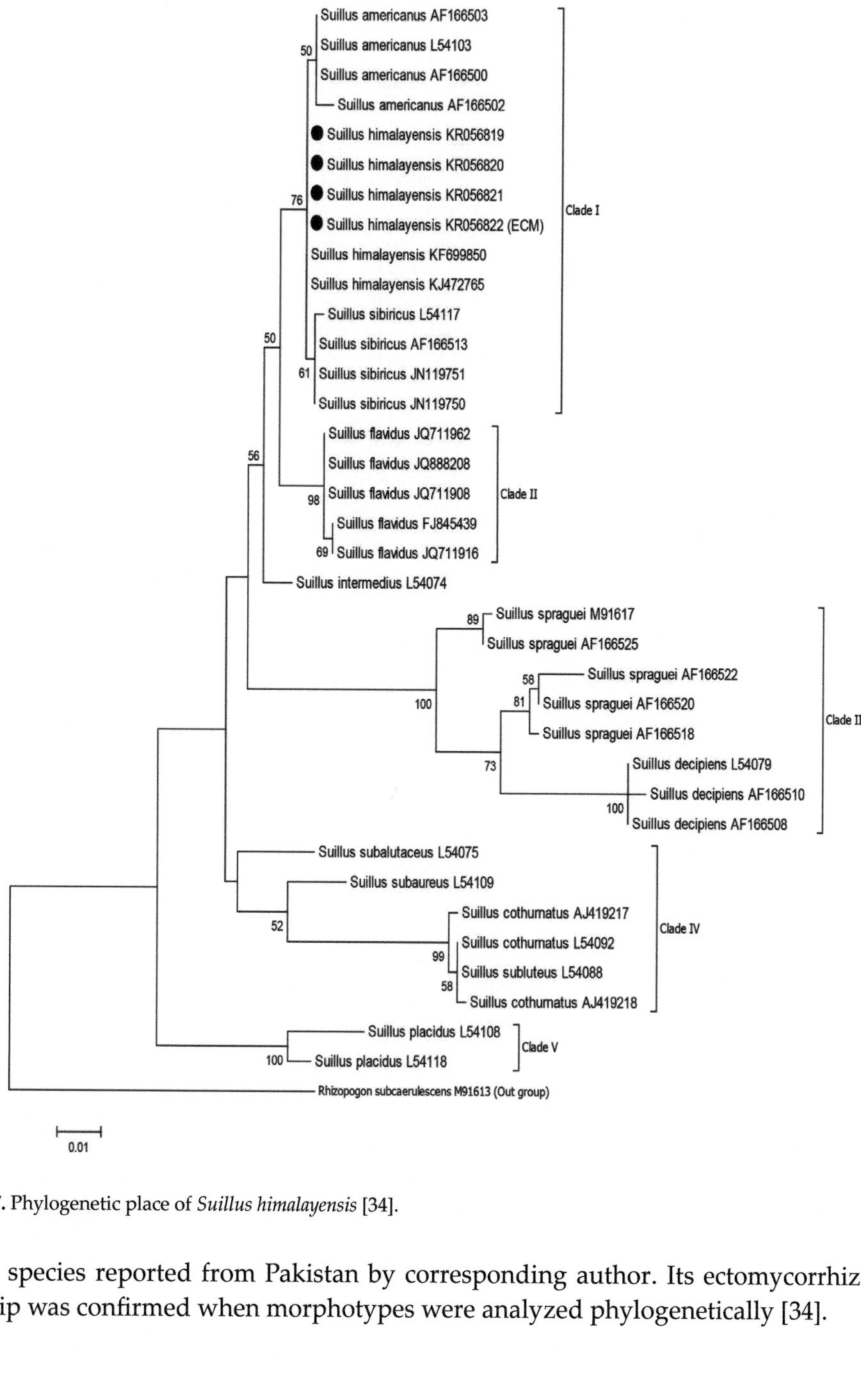

Figure 7. Phylogenetic place of *Suillus himalayensis* [34].

a new species reported from Pakistan by corresponding author. Its ectomycorrhizal relationship was confirmed when morphotypes were analyzed phylogenetically [34].

5. Problems that need to be addressed

The absence of sequences at a local level would be a chief hindrance for the recognition of some Basidiomycetes. Robles et al. [35] worked to analyze the scope of facts attained from ITS sequences as taxonomic implements to inspect local wood-rotting fungi. Phylogenetic analyses were made under static and vibrant homologies, but identification of some of these fungi was not attained due to the intricacy of the genera and the deficit of sequences [35].

Another fungus *LeucoCalocybe mongolica* has application in food industry and atmosphere investigation, is a noteworthy unusual wild edible mushroom in Northeast Asia. Its genomic sequence is vital to be studied at genus and species level in taxonomic classification. Beyond that, there is limitation in further study by virtue of the way that transcriptomic and genomic information of *L. mongolica* lacked in the biological information database. For such investigation, the transcriptome information is accomplished by virtue of Illumina paired-end sequencing innovation [36].

For taxonomic identification of Basidiomycetes, the sequence of the ITS region is a superior molecular DNA barcode [37]. As most of the studies so far done to identify the fungal species has used primers (forward and reverse) against this most highly varied region to amplify. Most of the times partial rDNA sequences, including the Internal Transcribed Spacer I-5.8SrDNA-Internal Transcribed Spacer II, are used, and further phylogenetic assessments are made to see relationships between edible species of the Basidiomycetes. Polymorphism occurred due to insertion-deletion and point mutations throughout the ITS regions and can be clearly distinguished within genera as well as families [38].

5.1. Why practice molecular documents?

Today, virtually all evolutionary interactions are contingent from molecular sequence data. This is because:

- DNA is the congenital material;
- We can here and now effortlessly, hastily, economically, and dependably sequence genetic substantial;
- Sequences are extremely specific and are often facts rich.

Morphological lineages are also made where genetic lineages are not possible (e.g., in few fossil records), but they are not reliable as we discern that every now and then the similar morphological mannerism can ascend from manifold independent evolutionary lineages.

5.2. Stages

1. Start with a question; which is the identification of a basidiomycete at species or genus level.
2. Identify a model and parameters that could answer the question.

3. Collect sequence data that would help to answer the question.

4. Identify the orthologous sequences.

5. Align sequences.

6. Estimate tree and other parameters given the data and model.

7. Estimate the error associated with the tree and/or parameter estimates.

8. Does it answer your question?

5.3. Phylogenetic resources at EMBL-EBI

EMBL-EBI offers a range of tools and resources that are relevant to the field of phylogenetics:

- Ensembl fungi are a vast resource for fungal genome data.
- Ensembl genomes extends Ensembl across the tree of life, making genome data publically available for bacteria, plants, fungi, protists, and metazoa. This includes pre-computed alignments and orthologues.
- Ensembl compara offers pre-computed phylogenies for visualization and download.
- ClustalW2 Phylogeny is a basic tool for estimating evolutionary trees from multiple sequence alignments. It uses the Neighbor Joining method with the option of a very simple model of sequence evolution [39].
- EMBOSS Seqret is a file format conversion tool that can be useful at multiple stages of a phylogenetics workflow.

After performing the first initial BLAST, a phylogenetic tree is produced using different software, for example, different versions of MEGA and SYPRUS (**Figure 8**).

5.4. Explanation of the figure obtained by using MEGA 6 software for molecular characterization and phylogenetic analysis of *Coprinopsis* species

After morphoanatomical characterization of *Coprinopsis* species gathered from plain territories of Pakistan, it was considered for molecular affirmation. Sequence brought about 1070 bp of their ITS region. The sequence was gone intensive BLAST search. Introductory BLAST investigation indicated 99% match with *C. cinerea* (AB097562). In addition, comparative groupings were likewise incorporated into this phylogeny. The entire informational collection involves 32 nucleotide sequences comprising 701 positions. The phylogenetic tree for *Coprinopsis* with sequences from Genbank was separated in four clades. *Coprinopsis cinerea* (BIF S21) falls in Clade I in *Cinerea* section making bunched with other *C. cinerea* species of different countries.

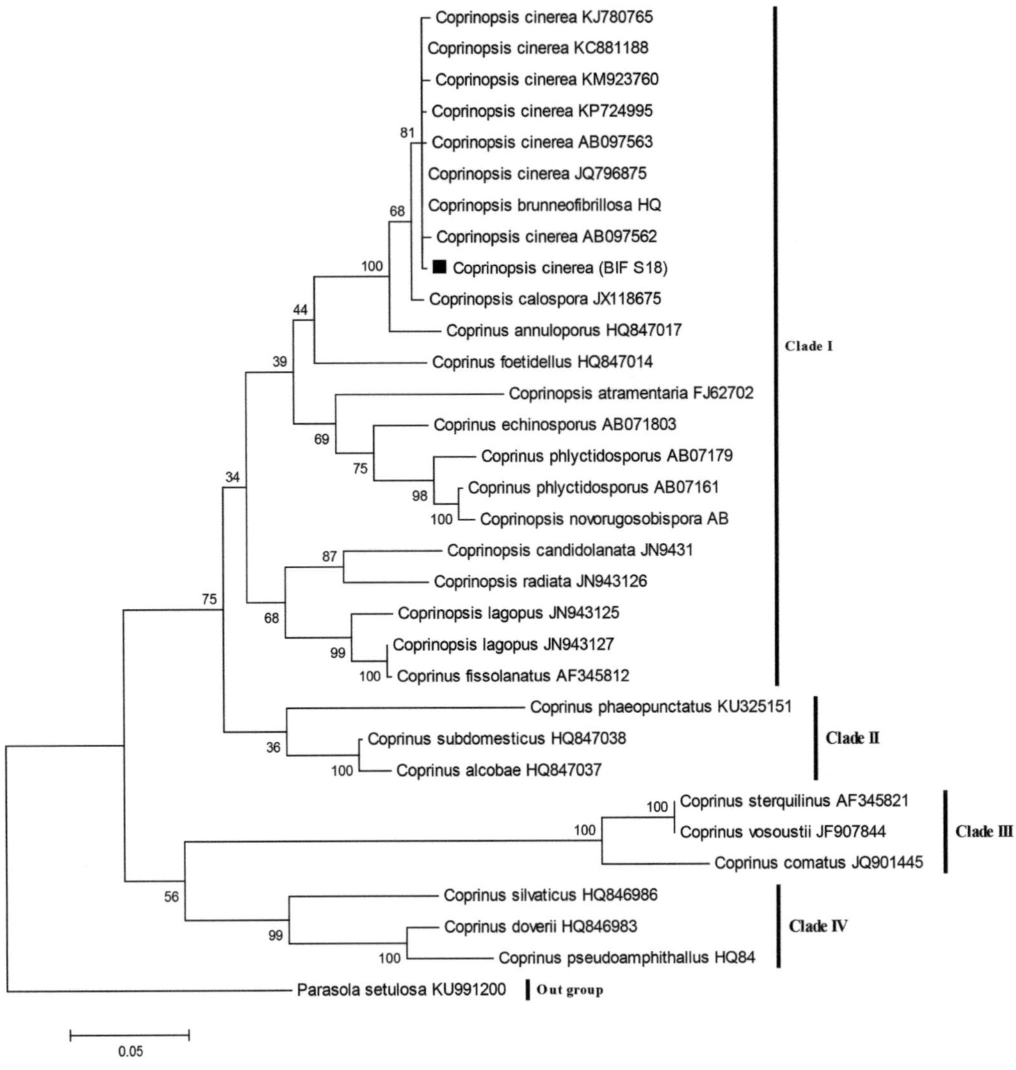

Figure 8. Phylogenetic analysis of Coprinus species collected from Pakistan based on nrITSr-DNA regions. This is the original phylogenetic tree made by one of the author of this chapter.

6. Conclusion

Basidiomycete is an important group of fungi that includes fungi forming ectomycorrhizae with trees, edible and medicinally important mushrooms, saprotrophs of wood and leaf litter, etc. and pathogens causing tree decline, wilting, and rots. Most of these have been identified and divided by morphological basis till eighteenth century by Friesian system, that is, all gilled fungi were included in Agaricales, all nongilled fungi in Aphyllophorales, and all macrofungi with internal spore production in Gasteromycetes. Molecular methods using DNA extraction, amplification of a specific target region, and sequencing have confirmed to be more steadfast methods of identification. Molecular and phylogenetic characters have

http://dx.doi.org/10.5772/intechopen.80671

resolved many controversies. Although classical methods are useful for enlisting species of a particular area, these methods for fungal identification alone cannot work better due to phenotypic variations. Combining classical approach with molecular and phylogenetic techniques is an appropriate way for identification, taxonomic, and purposes.

Author details

Samina Sarwar*, Qudsia Firdous and Abdul Nasir Khalid

*Address all correspondence to: samina_boletus@yahoo.com

Department of Botany, Lahore College for Women University, Lahore, Pakistan

References

[1] Hall AE, Fiebig A, Preuss D. Beyond the *Arabidopsis* genome: Opportunities for comparative genomics. Plant Physiology. 2002;**129**:1439-1447

[2] Doyle JJ, Luckow MS. The rest of the iceberg: Legume diversity and evolution in a phylogenetic context. Plant Physiology. 2003;**131**(3):900-910

[3] Fell JW, Boekhout T, Fonseca A, Sampaio JP. Basidiomycetous yeasts. In: Mclaughlin DJ, McLaughlin EG, Lemke PA, editors. The Mycota VII. Systematics and Evolution. Part B. Berlin: Springer-Verlag; 2001. pp. 1-36

[4] Nagy LG, Szöllősi G. Fungal phylogeny in the age of genomics: Insights into phylogenetic inference from genome-scale datasets. Advances in Genetics. 2017;**100**:49-72

[5] Floudas D, Held BW, Riley R, Nagy LG, Koehler G, Ransdell AS, et al. Evolution of novel wood decay mechanisms in Agaricales revealed by the genome sequences of *Fistulina hepatica* and *Cylindrobasidium torrendii*. Fungal Genetics and Biology. 2015;**76**:78-92

[6] Mueller GM, Schmit JP. Fungal biodiversity: What do we know? What can we predict? Biodiversity and Conservation. 2007;**16**(1):1-5

[7] O'Brien HE, Parrent JP, Jackson JA, Moncalvo JM, Vilgalys R. Fungal community analysis by large–scale sequencing of environmental samples. Applied and Environmental Microbiology. 2005;**71**(9):5544-5550

[8] Raghukumar S. Fungi: Characteristics and classification. In: Fungi in Coastal and Oceanic Marine Ecosystems. Cham: Springer; 2017. pp. 1-15

[9] Wołoszyn A, Kotłowski R. A universal method for the identification of genes encoding amatoxins and phallotoxins in poisonous mushrooms. Roczniki Panstwowego Zakladu Higieny. 2017;**68**(3):247-251

[10] Hawksworth DL. The magnitude of fungal diversity: The 1.5 million species revisited. Mycological Research. 2001;**105**:1422-1432

[11] Hood IA. Heart rot and root rot in tropical *Acacia* plantations. In: Potter K, Rimbawanto A, Beadle C, editors. Proceedings of a Workshop Held in Yogyakarta, Indonesia; 7-9 February 2006; Canberra, ACIAR Proceedings No. 124; The Mycology of the Basidiomycetes; 2006

[12] Govindaraj R, Paulraj MG, Ignacimuthu S. New record of *Mutinus caninus* (Huds.) Fr. (Phallaceae) in southern India, Tamil Nadu. Journal of Academia and Industrial Research. 2016;**4**(9):206

[13] Old KM, Lee SS, Sharma JK, Yuan ZQ. A Manual of Diseases of Tropical Acacias in Australia, SouthEast Asia and India. Jakarta, Indonesia: Centre for International Forestry Research; 2000. p. 104

[14] Zhao RL, Zhou JL, Chen J, Margaritescu S, Sanchez–Ramirez S, Hyde KD, et al. Towards standardizing taxonomic ranks using divergence times—A case study for reconstruction of the *Agaricus* taxonomic system. Fungal Diversity. 2016;**3**:1-54

[15] Shi C, Singh P, Ranieri ML, Wiedmann M, Switt AIM. Molecular methods for serovar determination of *Salmonella*. Critical Reviews in Microbiology. 2015;**41**(3):309-325

[16] Potter K, Rimbawanto A, Beadle C, editors. Heart rot and root rot in tropical *Acacia* plantations. In: Proceedings of a workshop held in Yogyakarta, Indonesia; 7-9 February 2006; Canberra, ACIAR Proceedings No. 124; 2006

[17] Kondo K, Nakamura K, Ishigaki T, Sakata K, Obitsu S, Noguchi A, et al. Molecular phylogenetic analysis of new *Entoloma rhodopolium*-related species in Japan and its identification method using PCR-RFLP. Scientific Reports. 2017;**7**(1):14942

[18] Aslam S, Tahir A, Aslam MF, Alam MW, Shedayi AA, Sadia S. Recent advances in molecular techniques for the identification of phytopathogenic fungi–A mini review. Journal of Plant Interactions. 2017;**12**(1):493-504

[19] Murray V. Improved double–stranded DNA sequencing using the linear polymerase chain reaction. Nucleic Acids Research. 1989;**17**(21):88-89

[20] Savard L, Li P, Strauss HS, Chase WM, Michaud M, Bousquet J. Chloroplast and nuclear gene sequences indicate late Pennsylvanian time for the last common ancestor of extant seed plants. Proceedings of the National Academy of Sciences of the United States of America. 1994;**91**:5163-5167

[21] Nilsson RH, Ryberg M, Kristiansson E, Abarenkov K, Larsson K-H, Kõljalg U. Taxonomic reliability of DNA sequences in public sequences databases: A fungal perspective. PLoS One. 2006;**1**:e59

[22] Goodwin CS, Armstrong JA, Chilvers T, Peters M, Collins MD, Sly L, et al. Transfer of *Campylobacter pylori* and *Campylobacter mustelae* to *Helicobacter* gen. nov. as *Helicobacter pylori* comb. nov. and *Helicobacter mustelae* comb. nov., respectively. International Journal of Systematic Bacteriology. 1989;**39**:397-405

[23] Garnica S, Riess K, Schön ME, Oberwinkler F, Setaro SD. Divergence times and phylogenetic patterns of Sebacinales, a highly diverse and widespread fungal lineage. PLoS One. 2016;**11**(3):e0149531

[24] Nawaz F, Jabeen S, Kahlid AN. New and noteworthy Melanoleuca (Pluteaceae) from Pakistan. Phytotaxa. 2017;**311**(2):175-184

[25] Bon M. Les Tricholomes et ressemblants. Flore mycologique d'Europe 5. Documents mycologiques. Mémoires hors-série. 1991;**2**:1-161

[26] Boekhout T. Melanoleuca Pat. In: Bas C et al., editors. Flora agaricina neerlandica. Vol. 4. Rotterdam/Brookfield: A.A. Balkema; 1999. pp. 153-165

[27] Vizzini A, Para R, Fontenla R, Ghignone S, Ercole E. A preliminary ITS phylogeny of Melanoleuca (Agaricales) with special reference to European taxa. Mycotaxon. 2011; **118**:361-381

[28] Agerer R. Characterization of ectomycorrhizae. In: Norris JR, Read DJ, Varma AK, editors. Methods in Microbiology: Techniques for the Study of Mycorrhiza. London, UK: Academic Press; 1991. pp. 25-73

[29] Mello AH, Antonioll ZI, Kaminski J, Souza EL, Oliveira VL. Arbuscular and ectomycorrhizal fungi in eucalypt cultivation and grassland sandy soil. Ciência Florestal. 2006; **16**:293-301

[30] Sarwar S, Hanif M, Khalid AN, Guinberteau J. Diversity of Boletes in Pakistan; focus on *Suillus brevipes* and *Suillus sibiricus*. In: Proceedings of the 7th International Conference on Mushroom Biology and Mushroom Products; 4-7 October; Arcachon: France. 2011;**1**: 123-133

[31] Hanif M, Khalid AN, Sarwar S. Additions to the Ectomycorrhizae associated with Himalayan Cedar (*Cedrus deodara*) using rDNA-ITS. International Journal of Agriculture and Biology. 2012;**13**:1062-1067

[32] Sarwar S, Khalid AN, Hanif M, Niazi AR. *Suillus flavidus* and its ectomycorrhizae with *Pinus wallichiana* in Pakistan. Mycotaxon. 2012;**12**:225-232

[33] Sarwar S. Boletes and their ectomycorrhizal morphotypes from some coniferous forests of Pakistan [PhD thesis]. Lahore, Pakistan: Deptt. of Botany, Univ. of Punjab; 2013

[34] Sarwar S, Saba M, Khalid AN, Dentinger BM. *Suillus himalayensis* (Boletales: Basidiomycota: Fungi) and its symbiotic association with roots of *Pinus wallichiana*, first report from coniferous forests of Pakistan. Journal of Animal and Plant Sciences. 2018;**28**(2):576-583

[35] Robles CA, Carmarán CC, Lopez SE. Screening of xylophagous fungi associated with *Platanus acerifolia* in urban landscapes: Biodiversity and potential biodeterioration. Landscape and Urban Planning. 2011;**100**:129-135

[36] Lu T, Bau T. De novo assembly and characterization of the transcriptome of a wild edible mushroom *Leucocalocybe mongolica* and identification of SSR markers. Biotechnology and Biotechnological Equipment. 2017;**31**(6):1148-1159

[37] Schocha CL, Seifertb KA, Huhndorfc S, Robertd V, Spougea JL, Levesqueb CA, et al. Nuclear ribosomal internal transcribed spacer (ITS) region as a universal DNA barcode marker for fungi. Proceedings of the National Academy of Sciences of the United States of America. 2012;**109**(16):6241-6246

[38] Avin FA, Bhassu S, Shin TY, Sabaratnam V. Molecular classification and phylogenetic relationships of selected edible *Basidiomycetes* species. Molecular Biology Reports. 2012; **39**(7):7355-7364

[39] Jukes TH, Cantor C. Evolution of protein molecules. In: Munro MN, editor. Mammalian Protein Metabolism. New York: Academic Press; 1969. pp. 21-132

Chapter 4

Genetic Diversity in Banana and Plantains Cultivars from Eastern DRC and Tanzania Using SSR and Morphological Markers, Their Phylogenetic Classification and Principal Components Analyses

Dowiya Benjamin Nzawele,
Antoine Kanyenga Lubolo, Paul M. Kusolwa,
Cornel L. Rweyemamu and Amon P. Maerere

Additional information is available at the end of the chapter

http://dx.doi.org/10.5772/intechopen.79922

Abstract

Bananas and plantains are edible and vegetatively propagated parthenocarpic species of the genus *Musa*. They are used as staple food, dessert and cash crop by more than hundred millions of people throughout the world. However, the crop is threatened by several pests and diseases in central and eastern Africa. One way of partly solving this problem is to have diploids which have desirable traits currently lacking in the AAA-Lujugira-Mutika subgroup. The study assessed through 21 microsatellite markers pairs the cladistic closeness of the diploid AA-Mshale accessions with AAA-Lujugira-Mutika with the purpose of inclusion in breeding programmes. Results showed that the eight studied accessions of AA-Mshale were different from each other. AA-Mshale malembo was fairly well established to be among the ancestor of Lujugira-Mutika, suggesting the determinism of its pollen viability and the level of resistance to pests for including in breeding programmes. The use of two pairs of microsatellites per chromosomes linkage group established the existence of alleles' deletion, recombination or non-annealing. The closeness among AA-Mshale and AAA-subgroups (Ibota, Gros Michel and Green Red) so far established through other techniques was confirmed. The results recommend the use of microsatellite markers, covering 11 linkage groups for cultivar identification and diversity study.

Keywords: *Musa*, AA-Mshale malembo, AAA-EAHB, clade, SSR markers

IntechOpen

© 2018 The Author(s). Licensee IntechOpen. This chapter is distributed under the terms of the Creative Commons Attribution License (http://creativecommons.org/licenses/by/3.0), which permits unrestricted use, distribution, and reproduction in any medium, provided the original work is properly cited.

1. Introduction

1.1. Background

Bananas and plantains are edible and vegetatively propagated parthenocarpic species of genus *Musa* belonging to the family *Musaceae* which according to Meng et al. [1] has wild seeded species native to South-East Asia. These seedless edible species are thought to have originated through intra- and interspecies crosses between *M. acuminata* Colla and *M. balbisiana* Colla, including some back crosses [2]. These species constitute a staple food, a key commercial crop and a major source of raw materials for both beverage and handicraft industries for hundred millions of people in the world. They include 20% of the population of the United Republic of Tanzania (URT), and its production promotes the country to be the second largest producer after Uganda in east Africa [3–5].

1.2. Problem statement and justification

The east African highland bananas (EAHBs) are currently threatened by several pests and diseases, which need diploid parents with farmers and other consumers' desirable traits for inclusion in the breeding programme [6]. The edible diploid landrace 'Mshale' (Mchare [7], AA genomic group) of URT was identified to be highly similar to *M. acuminata* spp. *malaccensis* cv. 'Pisang lilin'. Research using numerical taxonomy on AAA-EAHB genomic subgroup from Eastern DRC and Tanzania has shown certain level of relationship with 'Mshale malembo', suggesting that it is one of the ancestors [8, 9]. These observations were supported by Simmonds [7] and De Langhe et al. [10] but need to be confirmed at a molecular level. Such research has not yet been done and remains dearth for the inclusion of the Tanzania's landrace in breeding programme. Elsewhere, such research using the AFLP technique has been conducted by Ude et al. [11], on phylogenetic origin of AAA-Gros Michel and AAA-Yangambi km 5. The technique has shown that these cultivars have similar ancestors that have contributed to their development. In this respect, *M. acuminata* spp. *malaccensis* cv. 'Pisang lilin' was identified as a source of one of their genomes (A). This supported the use of landrace AA 'Paka' from Zanzibar in the improvement of 'Gros Michel' in Jamaïca [7, 10].

1.3. Hypothesis, technology justification and objective

AFLP technique shows a dominant mode of inheritance and hence constitutes its limiting factor for this study. On the other hand, research using SSR markers has confirmed these preceding findings [12]. Moreover, the fact that the genetic map has 11 linkage groups of Pisang lilin was also reported [13]. Therefore, the determination of identity and confirmation of the contribution of 'Mshale' in the AAA-EAHB using microsatellite markers determined from Pisang lilin could be a useful tool for the regeneration of subgroups escaping genetic erosion due to pests. This would constitute different scientific point of view from the current belief that AAA-EAHB comes from somaclonal variation [14]. The study aimed to establish the cladistic relationship of the banana landrace 'AA-Mshale' in AAA-EAHB which may constitute a way for reconstituting the EAHB through breeding.

2. Materials and methods

2.1. Plant materials

Cigar (unfurled) leaf samples from 25 accessions of bananas and plantains (**Table 1**) were collected from the existing banana gene bank in the Horticulture Unit of Sokoine University of Agriculture (SUA). The 25 accessions consisted of eight edible diploids (AA), nine, four and two triploids (AAA, AAB, ABB), two tetraploids (AAAA) genomic groups which were determined through numerical morpho-taxonomic classification [15]. Apart from the diploids and triploids AAA-EAHB subgroup, the other subgroups and genomic group were added as

No	Name of cultivars	Genomic group	Subgroup, clone set
01	Unyoya	ABB	Pisang Awak
02	Bokoboko	ABB	Bluggoe
03	Mzuzu	AAB	French Plantain
04	Ngego I	AAB	French Plantain
05	Ngego Halisi	AAB	French Plantain
06	Kisukari	AAB	Silk/Kamaramasengi
07	FHIA 17	AAAA	FHIA
08	FHIA 23	AAAA	FHIA
09	Bukoba	AAA	EAHB-Musakala, cooking type
10	Embwailuma	AAA	EAHB-Nakitembe, cooking type
11	Mwanjunjila	AAA	EAHB-Nfuuka, cooking type
12	Muhowe	AAA	EAHB-Nfuuka, beer type
13	Kimalindi fupi	AAA	Dwarf Cavendish
14	Jamaïca	AAA	Gros Michel
15	Yangambi km 5	AAA	Ibotabota (or 'Ibota' in short)
16	Mzungu mwekundu	AAA	Red/Green-Red
17	Mshale malembo	AA	Mshale
18	Mshale makyughu	AA	Mshale
19	Nshonwa mshale	AA	Mshale
20	Ndyali	AA	Mshale
21	King banana	AA	Wild diploid
22	Huti	AA	Mshale
23	Ilalyi	AA	Mshale
24	Ijihu	AA	Mshale
25	Green bell	AA	Mshale

Table 1. Cultivars used in molecular characterization using SSR markers.

control to verify the accuracy of the ancestry. The SUA *Musa* sp. germplasm was an *in situ* field conservation located in the plateau zone of Morogoro Urban District of Tanzania [5].

2.2. DNA extraction

The DNA of the 25 accessions (**Table 1**) was isolated using DNeasy Plant Mini Kit (Qiagen, USA; www.qiagen.com) following the manufacturer's instructions, quantified in 2% agarose gel (in 0.5 TBE electrophoresis buffer) and stained in 5 μg/ml of ethidium bromide solution. The DNA quality was checked by ensuring that the 260/280-nm values ranged between 1.4 and 2.2 using spectrophotometer [12]. The PCR was performed using a Gene Amp PCR system 2700 thermocycler (Applied Biosystems). Each reaction was carried out in a total volume of 20 μl, containing 10 ng of genomic DNA, 1.2 mM $MgCl_2$, 10 mM dNTPs, 0.2 μM of each primer, 1.25 U of Taq polymerase and 10x Go Taq flex buffer (New England Biolabs, Inc.). Twenty-one SSR primer pairs (**Table 2**) distributed across the 11 linkage groups were used. This SSR primer selection was done among established linkage groups covering banana genome [13]. During

SSR	Motif	LG	Forward primer (F) Reverse primer (R)	°C	bp
mMaCIR105	(CA)8,(CT)15	6	CATCCACTTGCTTTTCCA CTTCACGGCTTCCACA	52.0	264
mMaCIR114	(AC)7,(CT)28	8	GCAAGCCAAAGGGAA ACCAACAAAGAATGGTGTAA	50.0	222
mMaCIR115	(CA)2	11	CAAGAGACTACCACCGAAGA TGATTCTCACGACGTATGG	53.0	114
mMaCIR117	(TC)20	7	GTTTGTGGAATAAGTGGGAA ATGAGGGAGTTAGTGGTGG	53.0	214
mMaCIR119	(CA)9,(TA)6,(CA)5	10	TGAAAAGCAATCCAACCT ACCCTGAAATGTTTGTCTTT	51.0	395
mMaCIR168	(CA)7	10	GCACCAAACCAGTCCTAC CGTCTCAGTTGCCGTG	54.5	243
mMaCIR172	(CT)19	1	CAGCTAATGCCAAACCC CGACTTCGAGCGAGC	53.0	258
mMaCIR174	(AG)13	2	GAACCCACCTCCCTCTT TGGGATTCCTGAGTGCT	54.2	167
mMaCIR180	(CA)7	1	GCCTCAGCCTCATCATC CACCCACTCGACCCA	54.0	226
mMaCIR189	(CT)3,(CT)16	2	GGGAGGGCAGAGGAA GCCGAACTTGGTAATGTG	53.0	259
mMaCIR192	(TG)8	3	TGACCTAGCACAACGCA GCTTATGTTTCATCGCCTT	53.5	133

SSR	Motif	LG	Forward primer (F) Reverse primer (R)	°C	bp
mMaCIR210	(GA)3,(TG)12,(AG)5	7	GGAAGGTGGCATGAAAG TAACCTGATACCCATGTATTGA	52.0	319
mMaCIR228	(CT)18,(AC)7	5	CAAGCATGTTAGTTTGGGA AAGGTGCATCCAAGGG	52.0	197
mMaCIR241	(TC)20	3	GCTAAGCATCAAGTAGCCC ACGAACAAGCAATCAAAGTAG	53.0	297
mMaCIR256	(CA)7	4	TTGCGGGAAACTGCT GTTGCACTGCCCACTT	53.0	280
mMaCIR257	(CA)7	9	CTTTACCGAGTTGAGGG TCATATCAGAAGATAGCCAA	50.0	234
mMaCIR273	(TC)22,(CT)6	9	TGGTTGAAGATTCCCAT GATCAAGAGGTGACAAACC	50.0	211
mMaCIR274	(AC)11	5	TAGCTCTTTCAACACTCTCATC CTGGAGGCAGCGAAC	53.0	150
mMaCIR280	(TC)7,(AC)7	4	GGGTCCCTGTTGGCT TTGCAGATTAGGGTGGG	54.0	221
mMaCIR297	(TC)9,(AC)13,(CA)9	11	GAACTCGGATTGTTCCTTT AGGCTGATGGTAGCGAG	53.0	173
mMaCIR301	(TG)11	6	CATGATGTTTGAGTTTGC CTGGAAAGCAACACCG	50.0	166

Table 2. Primer sequences, SSR repeat motif, linkage groups (LG), theoretical annealing temperature (°C) and expected PCR product's size (bp).

amplifications, temperature cycling was conducted as follows: an initial denaturation step at 95°C for 5 min that was followed by 32 cycles of denaturation at 94°C for 1 min, annealing at each temperature as specified in **Table 2** per primer pair for 1 min, and extension (elongation) for 90 s at 72°C. A final extension was carried out at 72°C for 7 min. For gel electrophoresis, a 10-μl aliquot of each amplification reaction was separated at 100 V for 2 h, using 2% agarose gels (0.5× TBE buffer). Gel images were photographed under UV illumination to check for amplicon size and PCR specificity. Allele sizes were estimated against 2-Log DNA Ladder molecular size standards. All samples were run with three replications starting from DNA extraction to maintain the integrity of the sample.

2.3. Data analysis

Alleles (0, 1, 2, …) were scored from 21 SSR marker pairs in the 25 accessions and were used to build the phenetic and cladistic trees. The data were analyzed using Numerical Taxonomy and/or

Multivariate Analysis System package (NTSYSpc) version 2.1 (Exeter Software, Setauket, USA). The Manhattan method was used to assess similarity among the banana accessions. The genetic similarity matrices were then used to construct the dendrogram with unweighted pair group method with arithmetic mean (UPGMA) algorithms that employed the sequential, agglomerative, hierarchical and nested clustering procedure [16]. The cladistic kinship between accessions was determined based on neighbor joining coefficients using Dice dissimilarity coefficients (matrix using NTSYSpc 2.1. The scattered plot and accuracy of the trees were determined using principal component analysis (PCA) and cophenetic correlation method (from NTSYSpc 2.1). A two-way Mantel statistic test of 500 permutations was performed to get a cophenetic value.

3. Results and discussion

3.1. Results

3.1.1. Molecular/genetic relatedness among accessions

The coefficient of dissimilarity varied from 0.28 to 0.66, being <1 or 100% showing no duplication among accessions from the 21 loci covering 11 linkage groups used as shown in **Figure 1**. Hence, the eight accessions belonging to AA-Mshale group were found to be genetically different. The dendrogram (**Figure 1**) established two main clusters (A and B). In the first cluster (A), AAA-Lujugira-Mutika accessions ('Bukoba'/Musakala, 'Muhowe'/Beer (Mbidde) and 'Embwailuma'/Nakitembe) were clustered with the seven accessions of AA-Mshale ('Ndyali', 'Mshale makyughu', 'Ilalyi', 'Mshale malembo', 'Nshonwa mshale', 'Ijihu' and 'Huti'). They included the tie of AAAA-FHIA (17 and 23) accessions with 'Yangambi km 5' (AAA-Ibota), 'Mzungu mwekundu' (AAA-Green-red) and 'Green bell' (AAA-Cavendish). Whereas in the second cluster (B), six heterogenomic accessions named 'Kisukari' (AAB-Silk), 'Ngego I', 'Ngego Halisi' and 'Mzuzu' (AAB-French Plantain), 'Unyoya' and 'Bokoboko' (ABB) were tied to three homogenomic accessions (AAA) 'Jamaica' (Gros Michel), 'Kimalindi fupi' (Dwarf-Cavendish) and Mwanjunjila (EAHB having a yellow male bud). The accession 'King banana' (AA) was an outline.

The genetic variation causes were allelic deletion or non-annealing and heterozygosis. The mMaCIR168 primer showed allele deletion in cultivars 'Ndyali' and 'Mwanjunjila' (first one and third three after (left) Ladder, **Figure 2**), and mMaCIR189 showed heterozygosis in cultivars 'Mshale Makyughu', 'Ilalyi' and 'King banana' (first six, nine and second three after ladder) while both primers showed a homozygote allele in cultivar 'Mshale malembo' (the first number six after the ladder). Similarly, alleles' deletion (null alleles) was observed among 19 cultivars for primers mMaCIR117 and mMaCIR174. The alleles' sizes resemble those of Hippolyte et al. [13].

The observed mutation has negatively influenced the principal component analysis (PCA) that resulted in poor fit of the clustering analyses with a cophenetic coefficient of 0.72 from distance matrix and 0.67 from product-moment correlation matrix. Consequently, the variation has spread over the principal component (PC) so that the three first PCs cannot hold the maximum of the variation (**Figure 3**) and hence weakened the value of PIC (Polymorphism Information Content).

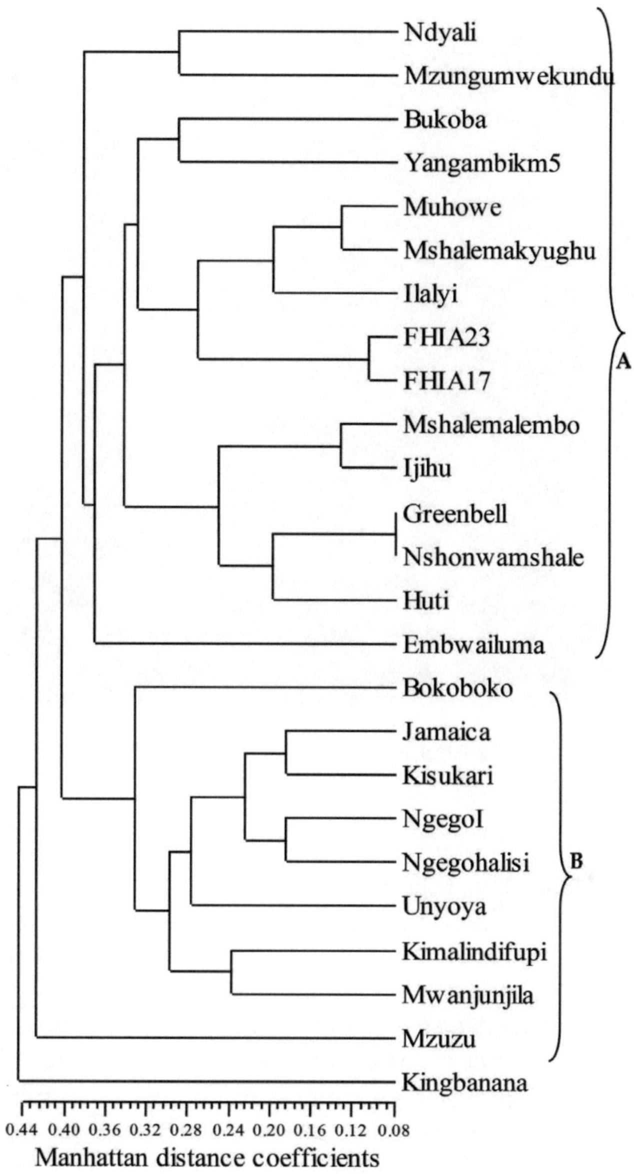

Figure 1. Phenogram from UPGMA clustering of the average Manhattan coefficients between the 25 *Musa* accessions using 21 microsatellite markers covering 11 linkage groups.

3.1.2. Cladistic relationship

The cladogram showed three clades which revealed mono-, para- and polyphyly (A, B and C, **Figure 4**). The eight AA-Mshale accessions were subdivided into two clades. The first clade (A) was a monophyletic group composed of eight accessions in which six belonged to AA-Mshale genomic group ('Ndyali', 'Mshale malembo', 'Ijihu', 'Nshonwa mshale', 'Huti' and 'King banana') and two of triploid ('Green bell' (AAA-Cavendish) and 'Mzungu mwekundu' (AAA-Green-red).

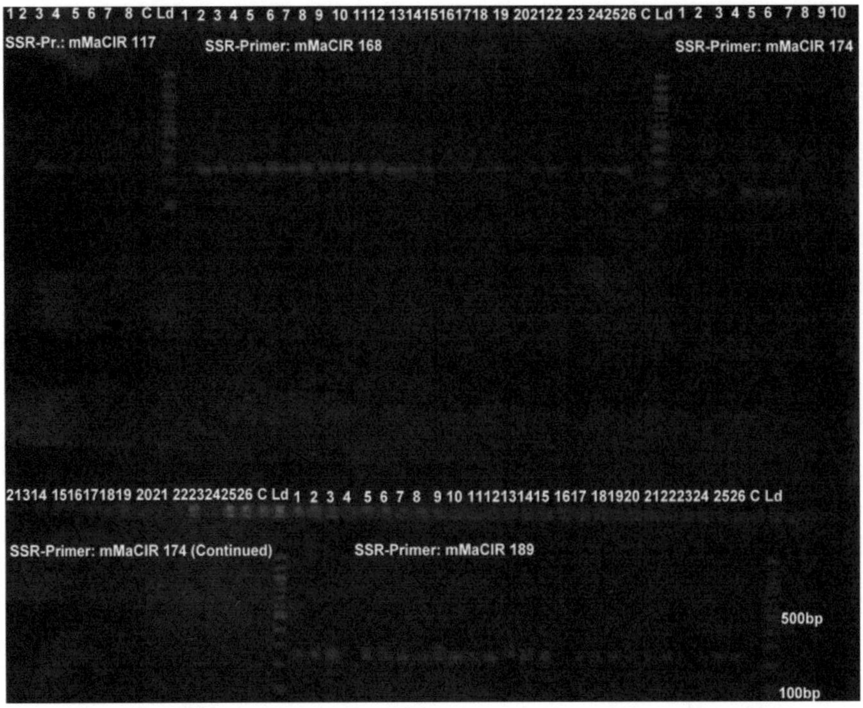

Figure 2. On gel image of alleles from mMaCIR117, mMaCIR168, mMaCIR174 and mMaCIR189 using 25 banana accessions (eight edibles diploids (AA-Mshale), nine AAA, two AAAA, four AAB and two ABB genomic groups) of (SUA) (Tanzania).

The second clade (B, **Figure 4**) that encompassed AAA-EAHB accessions was subdivided into two subclades (B1 and B2) and formed paraphyletic group with the first clade. The first subclade (B1) was made of three accessions, 'Mzuzu', 'Bukoba' and 'Yangambi km 5', that belonged to AAB-French Plantain, AAA-EAHB-Musakala and AAA-Ibota, respectively. Whereas, in the second subclade (B2), the AAA-EAHB accessions 'Muhowe' and 'Embwailuma' shared the ancestry with AA-Mshale (Mshale makyughu and Ilalyi) and AAAA-FHIA (17 and 23). The last clade (C) had 'Kimalindi fupi' (AAA-Cavendish), 'Mwanjunjila' (AAA-EAHB) and Jamaica (AAA-Gros Michel) sharing a common ancestry with AAB-Silk (Kisukari), AAB-French plantain (Ngego Halisi and Ngego I) and ABB (Bokoboko and Unyoya). The clade (C) established a polyphyly with the two first clade (A and B) that had AA genomic group accessions. Whereas, in reference to accession 'Jamaica', there was a paraphyly between the clades B and C.

3.2. Discussion

This clustering from dissimilarity using UPGMA fairly confirms the relationship established by numerical taxonomy between the AA-Mshale malembo and the AAA-Lujugira-Mutika group determined by several authors [2, 7–9]. Likewise, the observed alleles' differences among AA-Mshale accessions were in line with the morpho-taxonomic dissimilarity determined previously by the upcited authors. Moreover, the clone sets (Musakala, Nfuuka and Nakitembe) coined

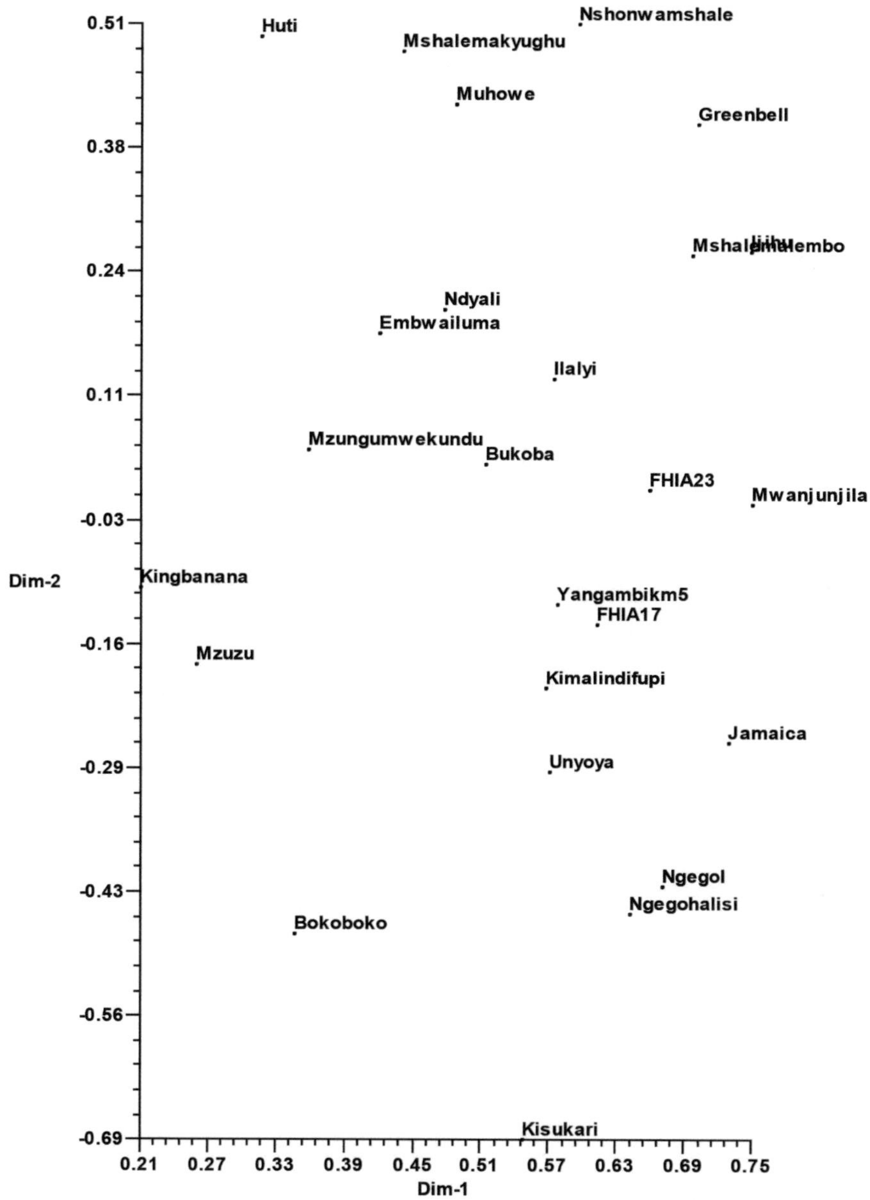

Figure 3. PCA showing the relative positions on the first (Dim-1) and second (Dim-2) PCs of the 25 banana accessions of the SUA's genebank using 21 microsatellite primers.

subjectively within the AAA-Lujugira-Mutika were linked with the different AA-Mshale accessions following their alleles' closeness [16]. Interestingly, the clustering of AAA-Cavendish, AAA-Gros-Michel, AAA-Ibota, AAB-Plantain and AAB-Silk subgroups as sympatric is similar to results of [11, 12, 17], while they used other techniques or primers partly covering the 11 linkage groups [13]. This once more established the usefulness and reliability of the alleles from the 11 linkage groups in diversity and cladistic study.

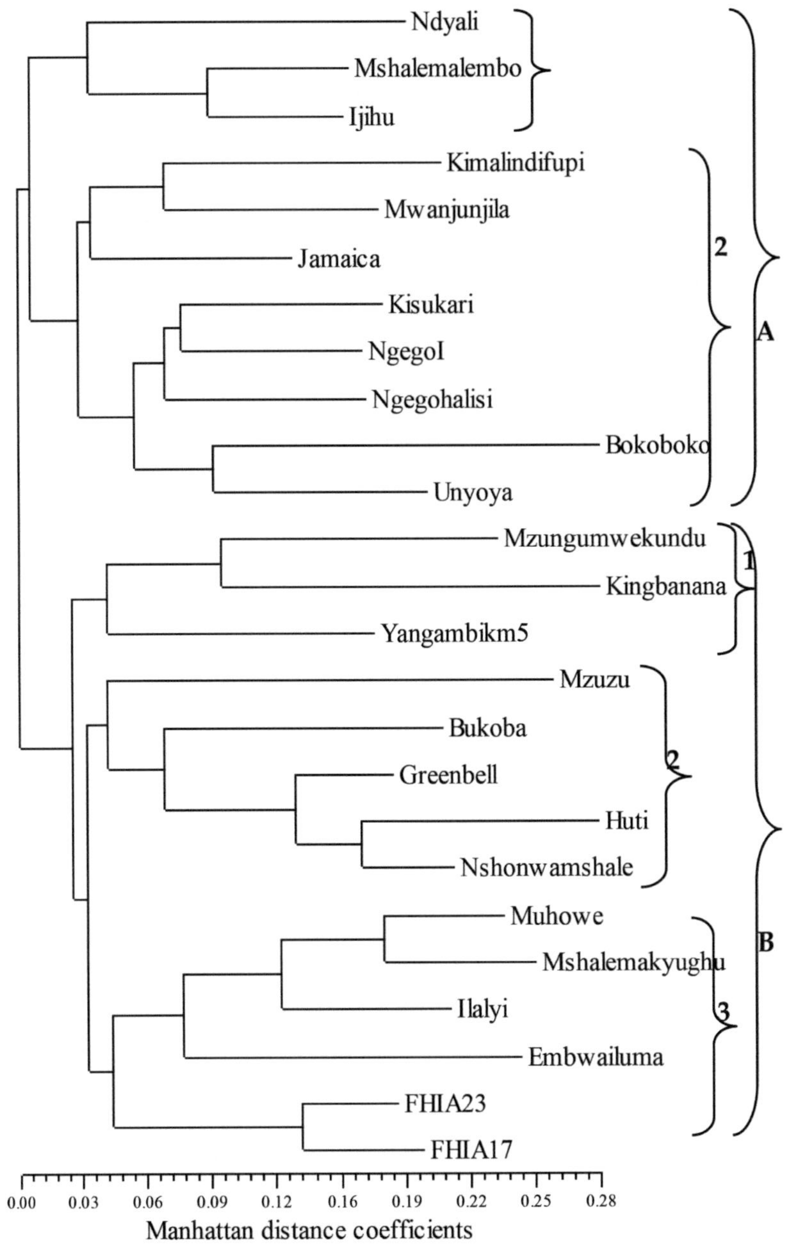

Figure 4. Cladogram from neighbor joining clustering of the Manhattan dissimilarity coefficients between the 25 *Musa* accessions from SUA genebank and 21 microsatellites.

The mono-, para- and polyphyletic relationships are in line with those revealed from numerical morpho-taxonomy [7–10]. The para- and polyphyletic relationship may be explained by the hypothesis of back-crosses developed [2]. The back-crosses theory explains the role of the observed alleles deletion and rearrangement (heterozygosis) in the evolution of AA-Mshale malembo in the AAA-EAHB. These relationships were also similar to results from other microsatellites covering 10

http://dx.doi.org/10.5772/intechopen.79922

linkage groups [17]. However, there is contrast with the statement of lack of convincing lineage between 'Mutika-Lujugira', 'Red', 'Ibota' and 'Plantain' subgroups, and the diploid *M. acuminata* accessions. This may be explained by the poor fit of the clustering analysis and the spread of principal components over the variables due to observed mutation.

4. Conclusion and suggestion

The eight accessions of AA-Mshale were determined at allele level to be different from each other. The contribution of accession AA-Mshale malembo in the ancestry of AAA-Lujugira-Mutika has been ascertained using simple sequence repeat tandem (SSR) markers. This suggests more studies on the parameters like pollen viability, germination and level of resistance to diseases and pests before inclusion in the breeding programme. The SSR markers constitute the best tool for cultivar phylogenetic identification, marker-assisted selection and diversity study.

Acknowledgements

The authors would like to thank the Canadian International Development Agency (CIDA) (through Bioscience in East and Central Africa Network/NEPAD) for funding this research.

Conflict of interest

The authors certify that they have NO affiliations with or involvement in any organization or entity with any financial interest (such as honoraria; educational grants; participation in speakers' bureaus; membership, employment, consultancies, stock ownership, or other equity interest; and expert testimony or patent-licensing arrangements), or non-financial interest (such as personal or professional relationships, affiliations, knowledge or beliefs) in the subject matter or materials discussed in this chapter.

Author details

Dowiya Benjamin Nzawele[1,3]*, Antoine Kanyenga Lubolo[2], Paul M. Kusolwa[3], Cornel L. Rweyemamu[3] and Amon P. Maerere[3]

*Address all correspondence to: b.nzaweledowiya@gmail.com

1 Faculty Institute of Agronomics Sciences of Yangambi, IFA-Yangambi, Kisangani, DR Congo

2 Harvest Plus, CIAT, Bukavu, DR Congo

3 Faculty of Agriculture, Department of Crop Science and Production, Sokoine University of Agriculture, Morogoro, Tanzania

References

[1] Meng L, Gao X, Chen J, Martin K. Spatial and temporal effects on seed dispersal and seed predation of *Musa acuminata* in Yunnan, China. Integrative Zoology. 2012;**7**:30-40

[2] De Langhe E, Hřibová E, Carpentier S, Doležel J, Swennen R. Did backcrossing contribute to the origin of hybrid edible bananas? Annals of Botany. 2010;**106**:849-857

[3] Evers G. Banana cultivar diversity in the area of Morogoro, Tanzania. Fruits. 1992;**47**(3): 377-391

[4] Msogoya TJ. Characteristics and mechanisms of in vitro induced variation in landraces of East African Highland Bananas (Musa AAA EA) [PhD Thesis]. University of Essex; 2007

[5] Maerere AP, Msogoya TJ, Mgembe ER, Mwaitulo S, Mtui HD, Mbilinyi L. Comparison of yield performance of improved and local banana (Musa) cultivars in Eastern zone of Tanzania. In: Batamuzi EK et al. editor. Proceedings of the Fourth Annual PANTIL Scientific Conference; 19–21, October 2009; Morogoro, Tanzania. 2010. pp. 172-177

[6] Beed F, Dubois T, Markham R. A strategy for banana research and development in Africa. In: Moorhead A, editor. Scripta Horticuturae. Vol. 12. 2012. [internet]. Available from: http://www.actahort.org/chronica/pdf/sh_12.pdf. [Accessed: 2018/ 01/ 02] ISSN:1813-9205. ISBN: 978 90 6605 664 0

[7] Simmonds NW. Bananas. In: Tropical Agriculture Series. UK: Longman Group Ltd. Essex. 1982. pp. 76-129

[8] Nzawele D. Distribution and genetic variation of eastern Democratic Republic of Congo's Musa spp. Colla and their relatedness with those in Tanzania [PhD Thesis]. Sokoine University of Agriculture; 2012

[9] Nzawele DB, Rweyemamu CL, Maerere AP. Genetic diversity among INERA-Mulungu (DR Congo) Musa spp. germplasm and their relatedness to those in Tanzania using numerical taxonomy. Plant Genetic Resources: Characterization and Utilization. 2013; **11**(1):50-61

[10] De Langhe E, Karamura D, Mbwana A. Tanzania Musa Expedition 2001. Rome: INIBAP/ IPGRI, Future Harvest; 2001. 107 pp

[11] Ude G, Pillay M, Nwakanma D, Tenkouano A. Genetic diversity in *Musa acuminata* Colla and *Musa balbisiana* Colla and some of their natural hybrids using AFLP markers. Theoretical and Applied Genetics. 2002;**104**:1246-1252

[12] Onyango M, Haymer D, Keeley S, Manshardt R. Analysis of genetic diversity and relationships in East African 'Apple Banana' (AAB genome) and 'Muraru' (AA genome) dessert bananas using microsatellite markers. Acta Horticulturae. 2010;**879**:623-636

[13] Hippolyte I, Bakry F, Seguin M, Gardes L, Rivallan R, Risterucci A, Jenny C, Perrier X, Carreel F, Argout X, Piffanelli P, Khan IA, Miller RNG, Pappas GJ, Mbéguié-A-Mbéguié D,

Matsumoto T, De Bernardinis V, Huttner E, Kilian A Baurens F, D'Hont A, Cote F, Courtois B, Glaszmann J. A saturated SSR/DArT linkage map of *Musa acuminata* addressing genome rearrangements among bananas. BMC Plant Biology. 2010;**10**:65-82

[14] Stover RH, Simmonds NW. Bananas. Tropical Agriculture Series. 3rd ed. London: Longman Scientific & Technical; 1991. pp. 15-425

[15] Sneath PHA, Sokal RR. Numerical Taxonomy: The Principles and Practice of Numerical Classification. San Francisco: Freeman, WH and Company; 1973. pp. 5-490

[16] Karamura D. Numerical taxonomic studies of the East African Highland Bananas (Musa AAA-East African) in Uganda [PhD Thesis]. University of Reading; 1999

[17] Hippolyte I, Jenny C, Gardes L, Bakry F, Rivallan R, Pomies V, Cubry P, Tomekpe K, Risterucci AM, Roux N, Rouard M, Arnaud E, Kolesnikova-Allen M, Perrier X. Foundation characteristics of edible Musa triploids revealed from allelic distribution of SSR markers. Annals of Botany. 2012;**109**:937-951